Portable Surgical Mentor

Portable Surgical Mentor
*A Handbook of Protocol for Interns
and Residents in Surgery*

Larry D. Florman, M.D.

Foreword by Hiram C. Polk, Jr., M.D.

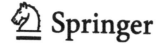 Springer

Larry D. Florman, M. D.
Assistant Professor, Division of Plastic Surgery
Department of Surgery, School of Medicine
University of Louisville, Health Sciences Center
700 Children's Foundation Building
601 South Floyd Street
Louisville, KY 40202
surgicalmentors@prodigy.net

Library of Congress Control Number: 2005926815

ISBN-10: 0-387-26139-7
ISBN-13: 978-0387-26139-3

Additional material to this book can be downloaded from http://extras.springer.com

Printed on acid-free paper.

(SP/EB)

9 8 7 6 5 4 3 2 1

springeronline.com

*To Sadie, Phyllis, Tammy, Jeffrey,
and Sandy, my mentors for eternity*

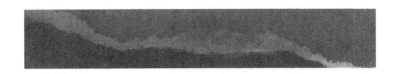

The Author

Larry D. Florman, M.D., was born and reared in Pittsburgh, Pennsylvania. He attended undergraduate school at The Youngstown University in Ohio and medical school at the University of Louvain in Belgium. Dr. Florman completed his rotating internship at the Queen Elizabeth Hospital in Montreal; general surgery residency at the Beth Israel Medical Center in New York City; and residency in otolaryngology at the Manhattan Eye, Ear, and Throat Hospital in New York City. This was followed by a residency in plastic and reconstructive surgery at the University of Louisville in Kentucky. He is a board certified Plastic and Reconstructive Surgeon, as well as Otolaryngology–Head and Neck Surgeon.

In 2002, after 28 years of private practice and teaching as a clinical instructor, Dr. Florman ended his private practice in the traditional sense and assumed the title of Assistant Professor of Surgery at the University of Louisville School of Medicine, where he has been training young surgeons to be plastic surgeons. He now limits his private practice to aesthetic surgery of the nose.

Acknowledgments

To acknowledge a few would be a disservice to all those who gave themselves so willingly and enthusiastically toward the completion of this book. But, I must do this disservice in order to emphasize the wonderful contributions of the following people:

Hiram C. Polk, Jr., M.D., for his constant concern, encouragement, and flawless expertise.

Ms. Carlene L. Petty, a wonderful artist, for her superb caricatures.

Ms. Margaret A. Abby and Ms. Shirley Cook, for their encouragement and masterful editorial skills.

H. Stephan McGuire, M.D., for his advice. He is only months from being a mentoree and is already a mentor himself.

Morton L. Kasdan, M.D., a most cherished mentor and friend, for his advice.

Judy Florman, a writer's writer, for the finer points.

Bethanie Hammond, a 4th year medical student, and the best mentoree a mentor could wish for.

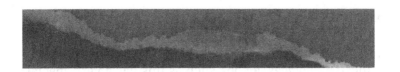

Foreword

Y2K may have been overrated in terms of its immediate disruptive impact on medical and surgical practice, but it also may have coincidentally marked an era of unprecedented change, especially in the domain of surgical specialty education. Whether one chooses to identify this with training in the beginning of the third year of medical school or the completion of the 7th or 8th year of superspecialty training, many of the same issues and concerns apply. The transition from a scientifically oriented student to a real doctor is fraught with hazard and consumes hundreds of hours. The transition into becoming a real doctor is fueled, in many respects, by what most patients expect their doctors to be. This marvelous, concise book is aimed precisely at helping you smoothly bridge the gap between student and practitioner.

We have witnessed a decline in surgical career choices, but now a reversal of that decline is occurring with a renewed growth of interest in careers in all surgical specialties. Studies on workforce, or old-fashioned manpower as it were, continue to show that there is a growing demand for surgical specialty services in America. Depending on where you live, it may be highly specialty oriented or nearer to "old-fashioned" general surgery.

While the most dramatic of these issues are best understood in the traditional format of systematic training in surgery in the United States, many of these concerns are international and apply irrespective of national boundaries. In fact, as an example, with a steadily important portion of the American medical trainee population being educated overseas, a book such as this has a very special and renewed value. The core competencies mandated for training in all surgical specialties focus upon the following:

1. Patient Care
2. Medical Knowledge
3. Practice-Based Learning and Improvement
4. Interpersonal and Communication Skills
5. Professionalism
6. Systems-Based Practice

These competencies reflect not only the old order of wisdom, skill, and knowledge in patient care, but a new order related to communicating our understanding of the health system within which we work, especially the need for ongoing professionalism. In earlier years, professionalism was taught in a simple apprentice manner by observing other physicians who learned from *their* mentors across generations about the ethical, the courteous, the considerate, and the humane practice of medicine.

Because of many issues impacting surgical training, particularly the shortened duty hours, opportunities for this type of observed interaction are now significantly less frequent; the nature of the American health system and its scheme for reimbursement has compacted the formerly leisurely, warm and personal opportunity that should mark each patient contact. It is ironic and also appropriate that professionalism to some degree is now going to be taught in a classroom and/or read in a book. One could find few better aids to crossing such an important chasm than this particular manual. Indeed, there is not a single anecdote or truism noted in this treatise that I have not observed, for better or worse, and would have wished to teach so clearly.

It is no accident that this is the product of a lifetime of experiences from an ethical surgical practice located in a hospital and associated with a major, old but characteristically mid-American school of medicine. There is no need to comment on such an overtly practical content, but communication involves direct personal interface with patients and all other health-care professionals. This is a reminder that "thank you" can always close any kind of contact with any of your professional and personal colleagues to your advantage.

The life of a surgeon involves communication throughout an evermore modern health-care system which, on occasion, becomes disruptive in and of itself. The surgeon's conduct in the operating room and in the office are special points of worthy attention, since they set the ambience for the conduct of the surgical team. There are now dramatic reports of the soothing role of teamwork in the surgical suite and those in which the stage is set for the highest quality surgical care with a minimum opportunity for adverse events for the patient's safety and well-being.

The doctor's office is another case in point, and the new surgeon should be reminded that timeliness is especially appreciated. If one does run late for very legitimate reasons, apologizing for your tardiness, and even offering to discount or eliminate the bill in the office always puts that kind of unpleasant interaction in a positive and generous light.

Despite the progressive growth of ambulatory surgery, the physician's participation in hospital rounds will continue to characterize our specialty. Again, one needs to be reminded that patients do not always hear and/or remember what you have said, and it may be helpful to clarify and expand some of these discussions, especially when concerning prognosis or directions after surgery. We should do this with another family member present and be certain to describe the nature of that discussion in the patient's chart.

"Compliance" has become a dirty word within medicine, but it simply means what most of us for multiple generations have known and accepted: write in the chart in a legible, accurate, and timely way exactly what you have done, what you have said, and what you expect as a result of that interaction. As a matter of fact, it may also be helpful to indicate what progress you expect in the period before your next set of rounds.

It has long been my thought that physicians who speak well, often think well, and being called upon to speak clearly and with a minimum of medical jargon reflects favorably on the doctor and all of his or her contacts. This especially includes presentations at rounds and in quality improvement conferences, which now characterize teamwork as a mark of contemporary medicine. Indeed, there was an era in which the solo practitioner was the prototype American physician. Now you are part of a team from the moment you begin your internship, often until you conclude your practice 35 years later, with the legitimate and ethical lifestyle of a hopefully closely knit group practice, defining exactly what one can do. The availability of a physician is essential, and one must never be less than vigilant in ensuring that your patients who are ill have the opportunity to reach you or a qualified and informed individual legally and ethically associated with you. The most difficult part of the 80-hour duty week, literally now in its infancy, has not been contriving schedules, identifying nurse practitioners, and/or creating night floats, but in the actual "hand off" a patient from doctor A to doctor B to doctor C. Everyone is alert to these issues that have posed unanticipated and unforeseen consequences, and we are all working toward methods to make those evermore safe and efficient.

The balance within one's life is an important undertaking, and this means refreshing your professionally fatigued mind and body with relationships with family and friends that renew you to resume your active surgical practice.

The fact that this book has been developed by a person with a lifetime success in practice who has now moved toward a full-time teaching role for new generations—not just for surgical specialists such as himself, but for the newest and least experienced third-year medical students—adds a layer of freshness, vitality, and interest. This book can be useful and will be the sort of thing that stays close in your hand and at your side across your early years in practice.

HIRAM C. POLK, Jr., M.D.
Ben A. Reid, Sr. Professor and Chair
Department of Surgery
University of Louisville
School of Medicine
Louisville, Kentucky

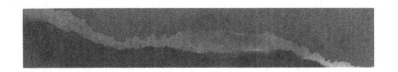

Preface

What lies behind us and what lies before us are small matters compared to what lies within us.

—RALPH WALDO EMERSON

This book has been lovingly written to aid our young colleagues, who by their choice of pursuing training in surgery have, in fact, dedicated the rest of their lives to compassion, study, knowledge, and humanity. The purpose of this book is to inculcate the discipline necessary for them to successfully care for the surgical patient and to teach this discipline to others. This is not a medical book *per se*. The subject may at first elude the young intern or resident. The principles will ultimately intertwine their lives so tightly that they will rapidly and joyfully witness in themselves the metamorphosis of the classroom student into the polished surgeon. My best regards and hopes for an exciting and rewarding journey.

LARRY D. FLORMAN, M.D.

Contents

The Transition

Part 1

> *My grandfather once told me that there were two kinds of people: those who do the work and those who take the credit. He told me to try to be in the first group; there was much less competition.*
>
> —INDIRA GANDHI

During the clinical years in medical school, you were gradually becoming a physician. Now you are an intern or resident. Veritably overnight, you must now devote your entire being to the profession that you have chosen. This part of your education can be very daunting, and if not taken seriously, can affect the rest of your career or even put a sudden stop to it. Whether you like it or not, once you received that diploma, and your family and friends addressed you as "doctor," your life changed forever.

There are certain conventions by which you must now abide. You must permit your education, your experiences, graduation day, and the rest of your career to blend in seamlessly with this new life. You are now a physician with all of the powerful properties and attributes that accompany the title. Do not resist your new level. Do not rebel against it. Do not believe for one moment that things will be the same in your life. Rise to the occasion.

Here are several guidelines to live by, and live by them you must:

1. You now LIVE IN A GLASS HOUSE

Get used to it quickly. Your every action will be noted and scrutinized by family, friends, and the public. Curtains on the windows will not shield you from the prying eye. The person who sees you do something foolish (or courageous) today may be your patient, car mechanic, or banker tomorrow.

If you have had one too many margaritas at a party last night, might not someone believe that you will be a menace in the operating room tomorrow? If you smoked something illegal, might not a close friend in need of you in the emergency room, question whether you had a little puff before coming to sew up his child?

How about the waiter to whom you acted like a positive jerk, and whose sister works in housekeeping at the hospital, and also whose brother cuts the grass for your chairman?

Your entire life is an open book, whether you like it or not. News of misguided behavior travels fast and is often quickly exaggerated. It is just about impossible to extract yourself from it. Make your behavior something you would wish upon your children.

2. BE HUMBLE

You have earned the privilege of being a physician. You now have achieved an expertise that very few enjoy.

Being a physician does not necessarily mean that you are a better person than others, that you deserve special consideration, or that you are higher on the evolutionary scale.

Each of us are travelers on the same road of life. If you are a better physician, then there is a better nurse, trash collector, or policeman. Only allow your pride to guide you to be the best that you can be, not to be better than anyone else. Consider the following true story:

I consider myself a humble person. I recently attended a high school reunion. I joined a small crowd having drinks. Many recognized me, and I recognized very few of them. As everybody was taking turns telling of their achievements in life, it came around to me.

"So, what do you do?"

I gave my usual retort, "I work in a hospital."

"Well, what do you do in the hospital?"

"I work in surgery."

"Well, exactly what do you do in surgery?" asked another of my old classmates, expecting me to say that I cleaned the floors or changed the light bulbs. After hearing of the multitude of successes of this small group—lawyers, businessmen, psychologists, internists—I said with a wry smirk,

"I am a plastic surgeon."

One said, "Yeah, sure!" The others bowed their heads, and the group immediately broke up and reassembled on the other side of the room.

3. BE RESPECTFUL and courteous to everyone that you encounter

It is better and easier to be respectful than to treat someone as though they were not there.

4. Be aware that MORALITY and ETHICS have a strong interplay when it comes to the practice of medicine

A lack of either may get you into the kind of trouble that could follow you for the rest of your life. Certain actions you take will change your life in a major, detrimental fashion:

- A felony conviction of any kind will most likely result in the permanent revocation of your license to practice medicine in every state in the US, or, at the very least, rejection by credentialing committees of hospitals and insurance companies.
- Any conviction for drug or alcohol use will most certainly result in relieving you of your training position, as well as your license to practice medicine. Retrieving either will be very difficult.
- Any lies, mistruths, or partial truths of any kind on your medical applications (training programs, hospitals, state license, insurance applications, licensing boards, etc.) will eventually surface and cause you grief for the rest of your career.
- It goes without saying that your moral values must be beyond reproach.

2

Attire

I'm tired of all this nonsense about beauty being only skin-deep. That's deep enough. What do you want, an adorable pancreas?

—JEAN KERR

Dress codes are institution-specific, which means that most institutions have a dress code, but it is usually non-specific. Dress nicely, appropriately, and professionally. Most likely you will begin your career by dressing very sharply, and you will certainly impress everyone, even your fellow slovenly dressed interns and residents (and some attendings). After a short period of time, you will see exactly what you can get away with, and in an effort to make your life easier, you will "sink" to the unwritten, house-staff invented, less than crisp, form of attire. A chief, attending, or hospital administrator would prefer nothing more than to see his or her house staff appearing very professional. This simply means a clean shirt or blouse, nice tie or simple jewelry, clean white coat, shined shoes (not clogs or sandals) and socks. Regardless of how your attendings and the chief are dressed, this is the way you should dress.

Dressing for your new station in life can often divert unwanted attention away from other inadequacies. Why not take every opportunity to impress your superiors? It does not take much effort, and it will reassure your patients

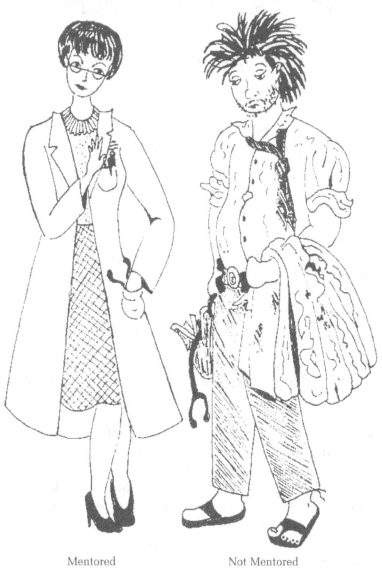

Mentored   Not Mentored

of your professional competence. You may even impress yourself with how well you clean up, and it could very well even start a positive trend among your fellow workers.

A word about grooming should not have to be said at this point, but we have seen too many ungroomed or poorly groomed house staff walking the hospital wards lately. This seems to be a holdover from medical school days. It is very noticeable and does not impress anyone. Comb your hair. Have your hair groomed regularly. If you have facial hair (beard, goatee, etc.), then it should appear neat. Better yet, do not wear it. Keep your face shaved. If you were on call the night before and must visit patients in the morning, then wake up 3 minutes earlier and shave. Get your teeth cleaned regularly; nobody likes to see your winning smile with a mouth full of tartar. Keep your fingernails trimmed and clean at all times. Patients and patient's families often pay attention to the fingernails of physicians, especially if that physician is a surgeon.

Scrubs should not be worn in the street. Some institutions turn a blind eye to this practice, and some absolutely forbid it. Not only does it raise the question of the cleanliness of the operating room environment, but you will actually start to walk into the operating room with those same street scrubs. Conversely, you could be accused of spreading hospital germs to the public on the street. It only takes one minute to change your clothes. For obvious reasons, do not wear scrubs at home. If you must walk out of the operating suite with scrubs on, you must wear a white lab coat. Never walk out of the operating room with a mask, cap, or booties. It does not impress anyone.

As mentioned previously, wear clean pants, clean shirt of any color, and (if you are male) a necktie in the hospital. A white lab coat is preferred; however, it must always be clean. Always wear socks. Absolutely no sandals are allowed. If you have been called to the chief's office, wear a blue or black blazer.

The same scrub rules apply to women in every instance. The same white lab coat, a skirt or a long dress is definitely acceptable in place of pants. A pants suit can take the place of a white lab coat. No visible body piercing, except for 1 or 2 ear piercings, and, of course, only those body piercings as mandated by religious customs.

You dressed well for your interview for this position. Consider every day of your life as an interview.

3

The Little Black Book

*Share everything...Play fair...Don't hit people...Put things back where you found them...**Clean up your own mess**...Don't take things that aren't yours...Say you're sorry when you hurt somebody...Wash your hands before you eat...Flush...Warm cookies and cold milk are good for you...etc.*

—From ROBERT FULGHUM,
All I Really Need to Know I Learned in Kindergarten

How often have you observed a more senior resident in his clean, pressed, white lab coat, with pens and little flash lights arranged neatly in his lapel pocket, tie precisely placed, stethoscope just peeking out so that everybody knows he is a doctor, and a bunch of crumpled papers hanging out of his pockets? Medicine is a rather orderly avocation, and any hint of disorganization gives the overall impression of confusion and sloppiness. A device that helps you organize your life and your job must be at your fingertips at all times.

In the past this method consisted of a little 6 or 8-ring "black book." While this is still used by some, the electronic substitute is rapidly taking over. Traditionally (and currently), the drug companies and other purveyors of medical items and services have made these available at no cost to the house staff. However, they usually do not fulfill the need.

This little black book, whether electronic or traditional, should be used to store the information about your life and your job in an orderly fashion, and at the same time, be easily accessible. Here are a few of the items that this portable medium must include:

- Calendar with as much detail as possible (meetings, schedules, rounds, holidays, vacations, birthdays, time off, deadlines, etc.)
- Names, addresses, and phone, cellular, pager, and fax numbers, as well as e-mail addresses of everyone you may possibly need to contact
- Phone numbers of various hospitals, with extension numbers of frequently used departments (operating room, scheduling, nursing units, medical records, medical staff office, emergency department, pathology, x-ray, lab, etc.)
- Patient lists (annotated)
- A section for frequently used drugs, their doses, and special indications
- A section dedicated to the idiosyncrasies of your attending staff
- An appendix with conversion charts (metric/British), formulas, etc.

It is essential to adopt a method for storing your affairs in some sort of orderly fashion. You may have 2 choices—a PDA (personal digital assistant) or a little ringed book (3, 4, or 8 rings). There are pros and cons for each:

PDA

Pros:

(a) Compact
(b) No pages to shuffle through or fall out

(c) Easily readable
(d) Calendar is very detailed (i.e., month, date, year, weekly, monthly, yearly)
(e) Can easily be downloaded to your PC
(f) Bulk information can be placed in PC and then downloaded to PDA
(g) Alarms
(h) Never becomes bulky
(i) Can include a cellular phone all-in-one
(j) Ability to transfer information from one PDA to another PDA (patient lists, schedules, etc.)
(k) Possibility of downloading ACLS/CPR references, case tracking software, PDR, digitized texts. Some hospitals are equipped to download patient lists, lab reports, etc.

Cons:

(a) Cost
(b) Important to backup the information to PC on a regular basis
(c) Learning curve
(d) Graffiti not always accurate
(e) Some actions may take longer to get to
(f) Need to remove stylus for many actions
(g) Need to change batteries or charge

Little Black Book

Pros:

(a) Inexpensive
(b) Easier and quicker to access and view different sections
(c) Place to put extraneous papers
(d) The pen is quicker than the stylus
(e) Blank pages can be torn out and given to others
(f) No batteries needed, and no downloads, and backup

(g) No limit on memory
(i) Easier to keep patient lists

Cons:

(a) Need something to write with
(b) Can get bulky
(c) Need to carry blank pages
(d) Pages can tear out
(e) No backup possible
(f) Not as "cool-looking" as PDA

Whatever method you decide, you should make optimal use of it. Do not be without it. Keep it up-to-date, rely on it, and use it. It will facilitate your life.

4

Communications

What we have here is a failure to communicate.

—From THE FILM *COOL HAND LUKE*

Speaking in the medical vernacular is important to effectively and succinctly communicate with your colleagues. This subject will be discussed in subsequent chapters. In the current chapter, the focus is on the methods that others can use to contact or communicate with you via overhead pages, pagers, cell phones, two-way radios, home telephones, and e-mails.

The availability of clear and immediate communication is very important to quality patient care, from the way that you appear to others, to the smooth operation of the institution. Answer all overhead pages immediately. Never be complacent while screening numbers on cell phones or pagers in order to determine the importance of the messages before answering them. The usual, frequent, benign call may be the one instance when it is a very urgent message. Frequently check the condition of your electronic device. Make sure the batteries are new. Know where spare batteries are located for immediate replacement. Charge your device every day, even if it has a 36-hour stand-by time. Frequently check that the ringer is turned on and is loud enough. If possible, have it ring and vibrate at the same time.

What follows is a review of the modern means of communications:

Overhead Page—Very Unreliable

Every hospital has an overhead paging system, but this form of communication is unreliable, as it does not reach certain areas of the hospital and is not always clearly audible. It usually does not work in the operating rooms, restrooms, on-call rooms, or patients' rooms. Therefore, do not count on it. Never ask anyone to page you overhead. If you receive an overhead page, you should check your pager or cell phone to ensure that the switch is turned on and the ringer is loud enough. Of course, respond immediately.

Digital or Numeric Pager—Very Reliable

Your institution will usually provide a pager for you at no cost. It will be the "monkey on your back" for at least the rest of your training. It is your duty and obligation to carry it with you, even when not on call. There is no telling when and where the boss (your chief, your mother, your spouse) may be looking for you.

In the operating room, you should place the device on a table and alert the circulating nurse where it is located and what to do with it. There are usually several pagers on the table, so put a label on your pager so that the nurse knows to whom it belongs.

Cell Phone—Very Reliable

This is, of course, the gold standard of communication. Many institutions provide cell phones to their house staff at no cost. Others demand them from the house staff and make you assume the cost. When not provided, many house staff will purchase one at their own expense, because it will make their lives easier. Regardless of who purchases one, make sure that you make good use of the special features such as the built-in phone book and speed dialing.

It is considered impolite to talk on your cell phone, while with groups of people in restaurants, theaters, elevators, and in patients' rooms. It is against the law (HIPAA) to speak of patients by name in front of the lay public.

Two-Way Radio

Some institutions provide this means of communication for certain physicians in strategic positions, such as for trauma surgeons, who must provide a quick response. Beware that the usable distance is short, and these instruments should not leave the hospital.

Home Telephone

Your home phone is not off limit to hospital business. Never put your home phone on "do not disturb." Never neglect answering the phone at any time or in any circumstance. Do not screen your calls. Have a phone extension at your bedside. List your home phone number at the hospital switchboard. Make sure that all of your colleagues have your telephone number, pager number, and cell phone number in their little black book (see Chapter 3). Remember that cell phone systems and pager systems do fail from time to time. You are obligated to always have a line of communications open to your colleagues and to the hospital.

This chapter would not be complete without a word about vacations and time away from home. It is essential that your senior resident knows how to reach you during your entire time in training. Leaving your phone number with the department secretary is necessary, but not good enough. A secretary does not work on the weekends or at night. If you will be away overnight or out of pager and cell phone range, an on-call house staff person must be able to reach you. Often you will know the patients best, which is why you can positively impact their care with your unique knowledge of their history.

E-Mail

E-mail is a wonderful mean by which you can communicate with your colleagues in either a casual or formal setting. It must be kept in mind that the Internet is not very secure. Patient information should not be transmitted by means of an unsecured e-mail message. This could be a violation of HIPAA laws. Never communicate medical information or instructions to a patient by e-mail. Keep in mind that e-mails can be discovered by courts of law.

In conclusion, answer all of your calls immediately. Easy for us to say, but in reality, it may be critical. There are special circumstances and solutions to the ever–occurring exceptions:

Situation	*Action*
Page of any kind *while in patient's room*	Politely excuse yourself and answer the page.
During *case presentation*	Pager and cell phone are set to vibrate.
	Better to give it to another person prior to your presentation.
	Quietly hand it to another person to answer for you.
Scrubbed in the *Operating Room*	Ask circulator to please answer your page and then say, **thank you!**
As an observer at *rounds*	Pager and cell phone should be set to vibrate. Sneak out. Call back very briefly.
In the *chief's office* for counseling	Give the pager or cell phone to a colleague who is waiting nearby or to the secretary.
While being berated by an *attending or chief resident*	Respectfully excuse yourself and answer the page immediately.

5

Surgery Suite Etiquette

Small opportunities are often the beginning of great enterprises.

—DEMOSTHENES

Demosthenes was a powerful orator of ancient Greece who captivated his audience despite a speech impediment. He taught himself to speak distinctly by talking with pebbles in his mouth. To strengthen his voice, he spoke over the roar of the waves at the seashore. Demosthenes had a "great enterprise" but a "small opportunity" to improve his speech impediment and achieve success. One great enterprise in surgery is to improve working relationships so that the operating suite can run more effectively. In this chapter, we will discuss scheduling procedures, preoperative activities, conduct in the operating room, and postoperative activities.

Scheduling

The operating room is your "kingdom," but you are the ruler of this domain only as long as your reputation upholds. So, why not protect and enhance your domain and your reputation before you are placed in authority? As the "crown prince," your reputation will be judged as to how you behave in the operating suite, and it all starts with scheduling. Sometimes scheduling is a function completed for you by others; however, quite often, you must schedule the procedure yourself. Whether the patients are from the clinic or private office, have elective or emergency surgeries, make every effort to schedule the procedure yourself. Do not assign this important function to a nurse or secretary. The advantages are enormous.

Start Time

You have the advantage of negotiating the starting time of the procedure if you schedule it yourself. The scheduler can hear from your own mouth the exact nature of the procedure (i.e., the urgency, the lack of urgency, the type, and quality of the personnel to be placed in the room), and by knowing you, can better determine how long the procedure will really take. You must realize that there are fast surgeons and there are slow surgeons. There are those of us who can be trusted to estimate time rather accurately, and there are those of us who will overestimate or usually underestimate times in an effort to inflate our own egos, or will just not know. If you (or your attending) are particularly slow, then honestly inform the scheduler that you will need more time to perform the procedure. Remember, you may fool the scheduler the first time, but not the second time. The second time the scheduler will remember you, and could set your start time to begin around 2:45 am for merely excising a small skin lesion.

Equipment and Supplies

By scheduling the procedure yourself, you have an opportunity to inform the scheduler precisely what equipment and supplies you will require. There is nothing wrong with being very specific. Have everything you need in the room before you start, so that you do not have to run the circulator ragged searching for a 6-0 nylon on a P-1 needle.

Personnel

You may have the opportunity to request specific personnel. This is particularly desirable if you can arrange it, but be careful not to offend others.

Working Relationships

Take advantage of the opportunity to develop a working relationship with the scheduler or scheduling department. There will always be special times when you need a really big favor. You may need to schedule a case a bit earlier in order to make your wedding anniversary an "event", instead of a "memory." Be polite, respectful, and honest. Try it, you will be pleased with the results.

Drawbacks

One of the drawbacks of scheduling procedures yourself is that you will have nobody to blame but yourself when things go wrong. Consider the following:

Schedule early.

Schedule honestly.

Identify yourself by name and service.

Schedule all of the various parts of the operation.

Make sure the scheduler knows the severity of the case.

Make sure the scheduler knows the proposed duration of the case.

Make sure the scheduler knows about any special equipment needs.

Place your attending's name first.
Be polite, succinct and respectful.
Say "thank you" before you hang up.

Preoperative Activities

Your efforts in the preoperative period will be noted by
your attendings and the nursing staff. This is certainly the
most important aspect of surgery for the junior house staff
member, as your superiors count on your thoroughness.
This period begins when the condition of the patient is
discerned and ends with the surgical intervention. It is
your job to be up-to-date on all aspects of your patient's
care, and to keep your superiors notified of any changes.
Expect calls from superiors at the most inconvenient
times, and be prepared to answer some very specific
questions. One faulty step at times will require ten positive ones to correct it.

Assume Responsibility

Many of these suggestions may not be your direct responsibility, but if not carried out properly, you are the one
who will pay the price. Once these routines are established, you will become very efficient at accomplishing
them. In fact, you can make a real difference from time to
time by assuming responsibility.

Notes and Orders

Review progress notes and nursing notes at least twice a
day. If a consultant has been asked to examine the patient,
continuously watch for his note and any follow-up notes.
Review the orders at least twice a day. Others may have
written orders for tests, and YOU must know the results.

Reports

Watch closely for addendums to x-ray results and pathology reports. These can be critical in the care of your patient.

Wounds

If a wound is involved, make sure that you examine it daily as well as just prior to surgery.

Communicate

Remind and brief the nursing staff of the impending surgery. If possible, discuss the surgery with the patient. If this has already been done by your superior, you should still ask the patient whether he or she has any questions. Certainly do not refute anything that any staff has told your patient without first checking with that staff person. Get a little personal with the patient. Ask whether there is anything that you can do to be of help. Discuss the surgery with the family if appropriate, but be ever cognizant of HIPAA rules.

Consent

Double check that the patient has given informed consent. Again, be careful that you do not refute or confuse anything that your superiors may have told the patient. Check that the "consent for surgery" has been properly signed and witnessed. Many surgeries have been canceled in the operating room because of an improperly executed consent.

Document

Document in the progress note that you obtained consent and whether there were any family members present. If necessary, dictate a short note outlining that you spoke to the patient about risks, benefits, and that everyone had an opportunity to ask questions.

This is a good time to remember to mark the patient. It is a JCAHO (Joint Commission on Accreditation of Hospitals) rule that all operative sites must be marked before the patient comes to the operating room. This simple but necessary procedure has drastically reduced the number of wrong-sided surgeries.

Prepare

If you have not already done so, review the nature of the patient's condition, the anatomy, and the finer points of the proposed surgery. Whether you are junior or senior, be sure you are up-to-date on the most current readings. Fortuitous occurrences have a way of happening. If you are the first year resident and the senior resident has to attend an emergency, you may be next in line to do the case with the attending.
BE PREPARED.
KNOW THE ANATOMY.

Operating Room Conduct

You will be judged by your peers, your superiors, your attendings, the operating personnel, and your patients, by your actions in the operating room. Bad actions will be noted and discussed *ad nauseum* by all. It is your reputation, and you should protect it with your every effort. Your good actions will be quietly noted but loudly passed on to others. You will gain the admiration or scorn by those who surround you and even those at a distance. Of course, this applies to everything you do in your training, but in the operating suite those bad and good actions are accentuated. The good actions will earn you praise from all, thus increasing your confidence.

You will note your fellow house staffers do many of the items outlined below, and you will be impressed by them. It should be your desire to do all of the things suggested here.

Prepare

Study the disease and the anatomy before entering the operating room suite. Be the "world expert." Read at least two recent articles in the literature and be ready to discuss them in the doctor's lounge, in the hallways, and over the operating table. Sometimes you will not have the opportunity to show what you know. Other times you will find the opportune time to interject your new knowledge. Your superiors will be pleased to tell their friends and colleagues about the great resident who works with them and who is always prepared. Study the operation long before entering the operating room. You should not be in the operating room without a thorough knowledge of the surgical anatomy and the operative technique.

Reports

It is essential to have all lab reports and original x-rays in the operating room. This is your job. These should be on the view box or on the computer. This is not the time to be fumbling for the correct x-rays.

Time

Always be in the operating suite early. Visit the patient in the holding area. Start times must be adhered to. In most, if not all hospitals, the start time is the "cut time." Do everything in your power to have the patient in the room in a timely fashion. Beg the nurses. Entice the anesthesiologist. Prod your attending. Remember, if your case is late in finishing, the case to follow will also be late. This is not the way to win friends. Holdups seem to cascade, delays become additive. You can make sure your patient is sent for from the hospital room early enough. Even though it may not be your job, you will feel very good if you can speed up the process.

Be Helpful

Ask the Circulator and scrub nurse what you can do to help. When they help, you should remember to say "thank you."

Music in the Operating Room

Gently demand that the room be as quiet as possible. One word about music in the operating room: If you have it, make it subdued. If the attending who is responsible for you in the operating room does not like music, then do not bring it into the room. If anybody in the room objects to the music, then turn it off. If the patient is awake, make the music calming, not rock and roll.

Stay Put

Once the patient is in the operating room, never leave until it is time to wash your hands. Stay with your patient. Talk to him. Touch him. Comfort him. This is an extremely difficult and stressful time for every patient, regardless of his bravado. Problems may occur during induction of anesthesia. Another pair of expert hands may be necessary. Your calm and reassuring demeanor is mandatory. Gently demand that the room be as quiet as possible. No extraneous conversation. The center of conversation must be the patient at all times. The patient expects it and does not want to hear about the great movie nurse Smith saw last night.

Be careful what you and others say in the operating room during general anesthesia. We have all heard stories about the supposedly anesthetized patient who heard every derogatory word the surgeon said during her operation.

Skin Prep

Somebody (you) must be present for the entire skin prep, closely observing for any break in sterile procedure. Just because a senior, very experienced nurse does the prep, this does not mean that it is correct.

Assume Responsibility

As you gain more responsibilities, there are several things that you can do to make surgery run smoother. Write down a list of your needed equipment and supplies, and give it to the circulator before the patient enters the operating room. Notify the staff about the patient's special needs so that they can comport themselves accordingly. Show the scrub nurse what instruments you believe should be on the Mayo stand and what instruments certainly will not be used. Tell the staff the "order" of the operation.

Scrubbing

Scrub your hands as you would want your surgeon to do for your operation. Proper etiquette dictates that if you are scrubbing with an attending, you should finish when he is finished. Attempt to scrub, gown, and glove, and help the scrub nurse drape the patient before your superiors enter the room. Never forget to positively identify the side and location of the proposed operation.

Assisting or Starting

If you are prepared in your knowledge of the technique and the anatomy, this is the correct time to ask your attending in a polite, humble way: "May I start"? He may very well respond affirmatively and permit you to do the entire operation.

Be Assertive

Depending on what your role is at the table (i.e., surgeon, first assistant, second assistant—fifth assistant), you may assume that physical position. Actually, why not presume that by some twist of fate the boss is going to give you the case. So, why not just assume the position of the surgeon, and see what transpires. Whether or not you are given the case, it demonstrates to others, that because of your preparation, you are willing and able to assume the title of "surgeon." Even if this bold technique fails, you will stand a good chance of being the first assistant. If applied correctly, the above suggestion will show others that you are definitely willing, able, knowledgeable, and certainly assertive, which are all good traits for a young aspiring surgeon.

There is nothing wrong with taking pre-emptive roles. If he or she is sewing, take a needle holder with suture and ask if you can sew also. Do not ask, and then take the needle holder. Take the needle holder, and then ask. If there is a bleeder that is staring at you, stop it. If you can expose something with a retractor, then move the retractor or get another one.

Make every attempt to anticipate the next three moves of the surgeon, the next instrument needed, the next suture needed, the type of bandage that will be used, and the situation of the next patient for the operating room.

Idiosyncrasies

Learn by experience the idiosyncrasies of each surgeon you work with. At the end of each procedure make a note in your little black book (see Chapter 3) about his likes and dislikes and refer to these notes before the next case. The note might include what kind of suture he or she likes, how many throws in his knots, the kind of dressing, the technique, the music in the operating room, his or her favorite discussion subject, etc. Check with the residents who preceded you in the service for their advice.

Finishing Up

The operation is not finished until the patient is in the recovery room. You place the bandage as instructed. You stay with the patient. You help lift the patient on to the recovery stretcher. You help wheel the patient to the recovery area. You give any special instructions to the recovery personnel.

Thank You

When leaving the operating room, sincerely thank each person individually. Shake the hand of the anesthetist. Thank the nurse for handing you the instruments, and your circulator for running to the basement for a cotton ball. Do not miss anybody. Do it even if you were holding the fifth retractor and did not get any blood on your gloves. Some of them will look at you hesitatingly. All of them will remember you and the small gesture of appreciation you gave them. It goes a very long way. Do this for the rest of your career.

Postoperative Activities

If you are given the responsibility of writing the post-op note and orders, you had better check with the surgeon for the exact title of the operation. This is very important for reimbursement and legal reasons. Make sure the recovery room personnel is comfortable with the written post-op orders and the patient's overall condition. You should frequently check with the recovery room to determine when the patient is transferred to the floor.

Although it may not be your job, you can certainly assure yourself that someone has spoken to the patient's family. It is a good practice to go to the waiting room with your attending or superior. The attending will appreciate the entourage, and you will learn the techniques of speaking to families.

Consider this experience as a lesson learned:

A middle-aged African-American woman was prone on the operating table being submitted to spine surgery. The surgeons were discussing last night's Passover meal. The surgery went well, except that they surgeons were operating on the wrong two disks. The next morning during routine rounds the surgeons asked the patient if everything was going well. She stated that she was not at all happy as she heard the entire conversation that took place during her surgery, that she was wide awake during the entire procedure, but couldn't move, and that she didn't like being called a "fat pig." When challenged by the surgeons, saying that was impossible, she said "then how do I now know the recipe for matza-ball soup?" Everybody was sued, including the surgeons, the nurses, the hospital, the anesthesiologists, and the manufacturer of the anesthesia equipment. Everybody lost and paid money.

6

The Clinics

*Give what you have. To someone, it may be better than you
dare think.*

—HENRY WADSWORTH LONGFELLOW
(1807–1882)

Institutional Clinics

The performance of each institutional clinic will differ by
title and by rules. In general, however, there are similari-
ties, regardless of institution, department, specialty, state,
or local rules. For instance, clinic patients should be
treated no differently from your private patients, whether
they are paying you for your advice and services, or not.
On the other hand, just as in private practice, you will
also encounter difficult individuals (see Chapter 8), or
have unusual problems in the clinics. All patients must
receive the best of care, even if you do not like the
patient. With the help of your attending physician, this
should not be a problem. Remember, you are in training
to be a surgeon, but the patient is not practicing to be ill.
They are counting on you to provide them the care that
they need.

An attending physician will be in-charge of the
clinic. Very often, he or she will be present during most,
if not all, of your time. Every patient must be discussed
with the physician. By experience, he or she is equipped

not only to teach you, but to "scope out" the occasional "red herring." Also, he or she is morally, ethically, and legally responsible for what occurs in your clinic. Be sure to tell the physician of your successes in treatment as well as your failures, and certainly all complications, no matter how trivial they may appear.

Since these are your private patients, you must be on time for your clinic, be appropriately dressed, and behave correctly. Appear and act as the doctor you would want to care for your mother. The nursing staff is very busy during clinic hours. Try not to make too many demands of them at this time, and if there is anything that you can do, then do it yourself.

Here are specific points that I believe are worth considering while you are in the clinic:

1. *Entering the Examining Room:*

   - Knock lightly on the examining room door before entering.
   - Greet your patient by title and last name. Children may be greeted by their first name.
   - Most patients will address you as doctor.
   - Be careful to know the rules for unescorted minors. The nurse should be familiar with the local rules. If not, consult with your attending.
   - Never enter an examining room with a female patient unless accompanied by a female nurse, or reverse the order for female physicians. This rule can be altered if a family member, close friend, significant other, or caregiver is present. Having these individuals in the examining room also takes some pressure off the patient to explain the reason for the visit, and allows another set of ears to listen to the doctor's comments and instructions.

- Be pleasant, interested, considerate, respectful, and thorough.

2. *Communicating with Patients:*

- Avoid jargon when talking to patients. They do not understand medical terms, slang, abbreviations, or initials. Even if they are very sophisticated, they will want to hear common, understandable language when it comes to their health.
- If there is a language barrier, then a translator must be present.

3. *Examining Referred Patients:*

- When seeing a patient in consultation who is referred from another physician or clinic, an attempt should be made to call that physician with your report. The minimum response should be to send him a copy of your history and physical examination and your plan for the future care of the patient. These items take a little longer to perform, but are always appreciated by the referring doctor. They will also generate more respect for you, your clinic, and your service, as well as more referrals.
- A word about "dumps": A "dump" might be considered a patient who is thrown upon you by another physician or clinic, for the purpose of getting rid of that patient. In reality, there is no such thing as a "dump." Each patient who is seen in your clinic deserves independent and appropriate care. A bad referral does not reflect on the patient, as much as it does on the referring doctor. Also, this occurrence provides you with the opportunity to be a star, a hero, and sometimes to make a diagnosis and/or a treatment that others may have missed.

4. *Observing the Patient:*

- Be ever vigilant of drug abuse in your patients.
- Watch for child abuse.
- Observe carefully the demeanor of the caregivers.
- Know what to do if you suspect something negative.

5. *Follow Up with the Patient:*

- If you promise to call a patient with any information, then you must call him at the appointed time. Put it in your "little black book" along with the phone number.
- Do not allow the nursing staff to make calls for you.
- Do not communicate with patients by e-mail. You cannot be sure they received the message.
- Remember, when calling a patient, speak to no one except the patient, or the person who is legally responsible (HIPAA).

6. *Exiting the Examining Room:*

- Never discharge a patient permanently from your clinic until his or her condition is completely resolved, or he has been appropriately referred to another health care provider. Once this has occurred, write in the chart the precise disposition of the patient and "return prn."
- Always offer the patient the ability to return to the clinic or to call you directly in case of any problem with their condition.

7. *Writing in the Patient's Chart:*

- Make sure that a patient's chart does not disappear into the system before you are able to write in it.

- Write all notes immediately following the visit.
- Request that your attending sign all charts contemporaneously.
- Do not remove charts from the clinic.

8. *Ending Each Clinic:*

- At the end of each clinic, look at each name on the clinic list, making sure nothing has been missed.
- Check the "no-shows" at the end of every clinic, and take appropriate action when necessary. If the nursing staff handles no-shows, then frequently check with the nursing staff. No-shows can get you into a lot of trouble.
- Any lab or imaging studies that are scheduled must be followed up by you in a very timely fashion. Write down the type of test in your "little black book," along with the phone number so that you can call the patient with the results.
- If you are the more senior resident at the clinic, you must be informed about every patient that your juniors examine, before those patients leave the clinic.

The Private Office

There are at least three scenarios in which you might find yourself in an attendings' private office. First, an attending surgeon may offer you the opportunity to spend time with him in his private practice. If he does, consider it an honor that he thinks so much of you that he is allowing you to not only be introduced to his private patients, but also to see how his office functions and to observe a portion of his personal life. Second, you may have a mandatory rotation in the private office. This should be considered a mandatory opportunity. Third, in a pinch, your attending may ask you to work in his private office to perform a small function such as to remove sutures, inspect a wound, or even to deliver lunch. Regardless of the reason, you must grasp these opportunities and treat them respectfully and gleefully, since the transition from the clinic to the private office is the beginning of your transition into the real world of private practice. Dress and groom immaculately. Be gracious, humorous, and courteous to the private office staff. Do not question the attending in front of his patient. In the examining room, stand straight with your hands out of your pockets, and do not lean against the wall.

These visits to the private office could ultimately become a type of interview for a job, or possibly the beginning of a dialogue for a partnership. Do not take lightly the importance of the office staff and their uncanny ability to sway their boss's opinion about everything from the brand of paper towels to buy to the kind of doctor they would want to have in *their* office.

7

Rounds

*If you get all the facts, your judgment can be right; if you
don't get all the facts, it can't be right.*

—Bernard M. Baruch

Every institution has its own definition of, and vocabu-
lary for, rounds. For the purpose of this book, we will
define rounds as the time when you regularly see
patients in the hospital. Every patient must be seen by
the resident (not just the student) at least once a day, and
the resident (not the student) must write a note in the
patient's chart. Most patients are seen more than once a
day. The first rounds of the day should occur prior to
scheduled surgery, lectures, conferences, and meetings.
This will indeed assure you of having to wake very early.
It will also assure you that the patient will not be distracted by breakfast, or that too many relatives or friends
will be present.

Proper writing in the patient's chart will be covered
elsewhere (see Chapter 9, Documentation). What follows
are just a few points about rounds that must become auto-
matic forevermore:

- Write patient notes immediately following the visit.
- Sign the chart, date it, and write down the time.
- Verbally tell the nurse of all orders in addition to
  writing them in the patient's chart.

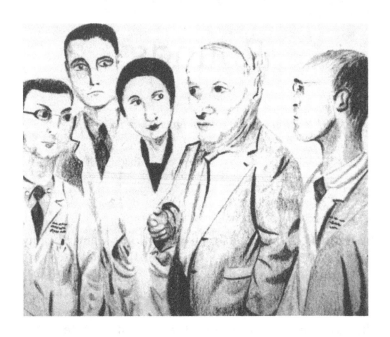

- If you are male, do not enter a female patient's room without a female nurse, or family member.
- Politely request that all extraneous visitors leave the patient's room, with the exception of one or two family members, if appropriate.
- Following rounds, seek out any family members, if appropriate.
- When with others on rounds:
  - Speak clearly and loud enough for everyone in your group to hear.
  - Use note cards.
  - Do not memorize a script; it sounds bad.

○ If you stumble, continue with a smile. Do not apologize for mispronounced words; attempt only once to correct it.

○ Try to anticipate all of the questions that you could be asked, and build the answers into your presentation. Do not guess at an answer. Do not make excuses for omissions in diagnoses or treatments. Never lie. Do not blame anybody for anything.

A few scenarios related to rounds

Rounds by Yourself

• If appropriate, introduce yourself, or remind the patient who you are.
• Dress appropriately (tie, pressed pants, pants and blouse, dress, clean white lab coat). (Flormanism: Dress like your mother would like to see you.)
• Apologize if you wake the patient.
• If you are male, arrange to have a female nurse with you if the patient is female (or the reverse in case of a female physician).
• If dressing changes are needed, the supplies should already be in the room, having been ordered by you the day before, so as not to waste time. Always think ahead.
• When you leave the room, assure the patient if and when you will return.

Rounds with Residents and/or Students

• If anyone is not dressed appropriately, send them to correct the problem(s).

- It is a good idea to have a more junior person go on rounds before you and undress the wound, if appropriate. If you are the more junior person, then offer to go ahead.
- Do not whisper to others in hope that the patient will not hear.
- Use medical language judiciously.
- Since anything that is said in the room with a negative connotation may be misunderstood by the patient, do not use innuendo, jargon, double entendres, or initials. Patients tend to perceive your every word in a very literal fashion.
- Be sure a fresh dressing is placed immediately. If the nurse is to do this, then ask the student or junior resident to check whether it is done.
- Be aware of sensitive issues concerning the patient, such as psychiatric problems, addictions, or family matters.

Rounds with Attendings

- Dress appropriately (tie, pants and blouse, dress, clean white lab coat). Make sure everyone else is appropriately dressed as well.
- Prior to rounds, the patient's dressings should be removed, wounds exposed and lightly covered.
- Any relevant imaging studies, or lab and pathology results should be available. Use note cards as needed.
- If your attending does not know the details of the patient, then make a formal presentation. If your attending is current on this patient, then only update him on the relevant changes.
- Do not permit any one to argue with or undermine the authority of the attending while in the patient's room.

- Nudge any discussion out of the room and into the hall, allowing everyone an opportunity to ask questions and make comments. This also tends to decrease anxiety in the patient.

Rounds with the Chief

- Dress appropriately, but do not necessarily dress like him. Wear a clean white coat and look fresh. No scrubs, unless the boss is wearing them. Anyone who is inappropriately dressed should be sent away, and make sure that this does not happen again.
- If this is a spur-of-the-moment visit, then someone should call ahead, and have the nurse or your junior resident undress the wound, ask the family members to leave the room, turn off the TV, and prepare the patient about what to expect when the boss joins rounds. If you are the junior, then do this yourself. Make your senior look good. He or she will remember you.
- Any description of the patient should be made on the way to the room, not inside the room.
- Be very brief, very succinct, and very clear.
- Always end your presentation with a plan for treatment.

Weekly Rounds

Each training program will approach weekly rounds differently. These are often held once a week, at the bedside, in an auditorium, or in a conference room, and involve many people, perhaps as many as thirty to fifty (the chief, attendings, residents, fellows, specialties, students, nursing,

ancillary personnel). This is your chance to excel or crash.
BE PREPARED.

If You Are the Presenter of Weekly Rounds

- Wear a clean white lab coat. Bring a pen, a
  flashlight (optional), and no papers hanging out
  of your pockets. Place the stethoscope in your
  pocket (or no stethoscope), but not around
  your neck.
- Shine your shoes.
- Get there early.
- Be very familiar with the patient's entire chart.
- Be familiar with what is not on the chart (social
  history).
- Be familiar with the patient's hospital course.
- Know all lab values of the patient.
- Have imaging films and reports available.
- Politely ask family members and others to wait in
  the waiting room.
- Turn off the patient's TV.
- Make a simple but detailed, computer-generated,
  bold-typed summary of the history, hospital course,
  operations, and time-line.
- Stand straight, hands out of the pockets, and
  maintain good eye contact with everyone in
  attendance.
- Address the crowd individually and as a group.
- No leaning against the wall. No looking at the floor
  or ceiling. Do not use too many abbreviations or
  initials. Keep your hands away from your face and
  mouth.
- Do not be cute.
- Speak very clearly; do not waste time with
  extraneous facts.

If You Are a Helper at Weekly Rounds

- Make the presenter's life easier during this really anxiety-laden period of time. He will do the same for you.
- Do his computer work, fetch and set-up the x-rays, turn off the TV, undress the wound and make it look pretty.
- Tell the patient what is about to happen and why.
- Support your senior in any way that you can.
- Physically and emotionally stand beside him.

If You Are a Listener at Weekly Rounds

- Comply with the same dress code.
- No secondary conversations.
- No chewing gum.
- Do not hesitate to ask questions. Avoid comments, unless addressed by an attending. **Look interested.**

Grand Rounds

Grand rounds are often held in an auditorium with many in attendance. In times gone by, these conferences would center on the presentation of a particular patient, followed by an in-depth presentation and discussion of the disease, and treatment with which the patient is presented. Now, these grand rounds usually are didactic sessions on a particular subject. They are often relegated to local or visiting experts. Very often, a senior resident will be asked to present. Needless to say, this is a very important hour for a resident, and needs much time for preparation and thought. Every point reviewed in this chapter should be adhered to.

Grand rounds are often attended by all the faculty as well as practitioners outside the institution. This makes the conference the "pride" of the department, proudly showing the best of their residents, and the active participation of the community surgeons.

Teaching and Teachers

This chapter on rounds is a good place to remind interns and residents in surgery that teaching and learning is the primary goal of your education, and the instillation of practical knowledge and technical skills is a learned function, taught by those who learned it just as you are learning from others. Regardless of your level of training, you are now the teacher and the student. You will be delighted to discover that teaching others is also an education for the teacher, a sort of learning twice. It is your privilege and duty to pass along your growing knowledge. Education in surgery demands the direct interactions between teacher and student, where both teacher and student depend on each other for their education.

It has been estimated that 40–50 percent of a resident's training is due to the efforts of fellow house staff. [1] Therefore, it is essential that interns and residents at all levels become good teachers. It is unfortunate that very little is taught to medical students, interns, and residents on the subject of teaching. Techniques for teaching effectively can be found in numerous resources.[2] References such as this superb little book will help you

[1] Brown, R. S., 1970. Staff Attitudes toward Teachings. *J. Med. Edu.* **45**, 156-158.
[2] Thomas, L., Schwenk, M.D., Neal Whitman, E.D., 1993. *Residents as Teachers: A Guide to Educational Practice*, University of Utah School of Medicine, Utah.

be not only the best teacher that you can be, but also, a better learner.

Note

Remember: medical knowledge is not proprietary. It is meant to be graciously shared. There is no need for residents and interns in surgery to compete. Everybody who performs well, performs well for the group. There are no bell-shaped curves for intern and resident prowess. You are judged on what you do and how well your group does. Do not compete with or against your colleagues. Have a burning desire for all to do well. It will make you look good to make them look good.

8

Difficult People

Kind words can be short and easy to speak, but their echoes are truly endless.

—MOTHER TERESA

Effectively dealing with the difficult person (i.e., patient, family member, co-resident, attending, consultant, hospital personnel) can almost be considered an art form, but this type of expertise neither can be taught as an exacting science, nor does it come naturally to most young doctors. It is learned from experience, maturity, and compassion. This knowledge must come very quickly, as the difficult person can enter your life when you least expect it, and can have a profound effect on you and the individual. The one saving grace about the difficult person is that you can often predict the difficulty before it occurs, so you should have time to figure out what to do prior to any misunderstanding or, better yet, prevent it from occurring in the first place.

The Difficult Patient

First, do not prejudge your patient. You may listen to others' evaluation of the patient, but it is far better to interact with him or her as though you are going to have an exemplary doctor/patient relationship from the start. If things go down hill from there, then you must critically evaluate the possible causes.

Was It You?

Ask yourself the following questions: Was your greeting incorrect? Were you not dressed and groomed appropriately? Did you not show appropriate respect? Were you too casual, and arrogant? Were you too "medical" and not "down-to-earth?" Could they read in your eyes and in your body movements that you might have lacked compassion, did not understand the problem, did not care, were in a hurry, or were preoccupied? Could they see by your questions and/or your examination that you did not have the necessary expertise to help them?

Remember, there is nothing more important to patients than their medical condition and their desire to return to health. This is all the patients think about, and this is all they want you to think about. Most patients are quite nervous when the doctor visits. They forget to mention certain things, and they forget to ask important questions. It is up to you to draw questions and answers out of them, and to be sure the patient is comfortable with you and understands what you are telling them. Go slowly. Be thorough. Be compassionate. Be respectful.

Was It Them?

Were they distracted by their condition, pain, not feeling well, and medications? Did something happen? A problem with another doctor? A problem with the nursing staff? A problem with family or at home? A problem with work? Angry at the world because they are sick? Angry that they are *not* sick? Lost hope? Do they have a psychiatric problem?

This is when all of your skills of understanding and patience come into play. These difficult patients must be converted into normal patients as expeditiously as possible. If there is a correctible issue (and there almost always is), then you must take the time and expend the energy to understand it, have the perseverance to investigate it, and have the compassion to make it right. Always remember that the patient is the real end point of your education and training. Do not fail the patient.

There is nothing wrong with involving others in assisting you with these problems. Psychiatrists, social workers, and nursing supervisors are most valuable in these situations and should be used liberally. It may come to pass that, even through your best efforts, you cannot succeed in getting through to the difficult patient. There may come a time when you will find it necessary to request assistance from a senior doctor, even perhaps the chief. Do not wait too long to do this, as the condition will grow worse rapidly.

Be sure to write the details of each encounter in the patient's chart. It is important to use exact quotations, and these should be documented with quotation marks.

The Difficult Family Member

First, be sure that you are dealing with a true family member or a person who is legally responsible for the patient. Do not forget HIPAA. When you are talking to a group of family members, you must identify each one in the group, and you must be sure that each person is comfortable with you speaking to the group.

Difficult family members can often be more challenging to handle than difficult patients. The same rules of conduct apply to them as to patients. Be respectful, understanding, and compassionate. Take as much time as needed to explain the patient's condition and treatment. Now is not the time for casualness. Answer each person's questions in a respectful way, even when the questions are inane or repetitive. A wonderful idea, even if not always practical, is to write down your name and a number (i.e., switchboard, pager number) and give it at least to the spokesperson of the group, by which they can reach you. Even if they do not use it, they will have a sense of security, and the definite knowledge that you are a doctor whom they want to care for their sick family member. It may even be advisable or necessary to involve the clergy, or the ethics committee of the hospital.

Be sure to write the details of each encounter in the patient's chart.

The Difficult Co-Resident

The difficult colleague is most often a fellow house staff person in any specialty. The problems you may have often fall into one of the following categories: work ethic, knowledge, attitude, general ethics, morality, and ego.

Unfortunately, you will often come in contact with individuals who violate one of the aforementioned categories, and this will offend you greatly. You did not ask to be placed with these individuals, but they profoundly affect you, your job, and often the quality of patient care. So, it is within your right and obligation to address and remedy the situation in any way that you are able. Very often, a quiet conversation with the colleague will make him aware that others notice his aberrant behavior, and he will attempt to improve. Sometimes a small group of associates who note the same problem can have the same discussion. If all attempts at mediating this colleague's poor behavior fail, as a last resort, a more senior doctor must be informed. The situation should not be permitted to smolder, as you will become more and more frustrated, and you will withdraw completely from the individual, which also does not make a comfortable work and study environment. Certainly, it is your obligation to follow this matter until it is resolved. Our profession does not well tolerate a deviant physician.

While we are on this subject, you could critically evaluate your own demeanor in an effort to determine whether you might be a difficult colleague.

The Difficult Attending

Difficult attendings can be a problem for every house staff member. Frankly, there is at least one in each department. Sometimes this person's less-than-exemplary behavior is directed toward one or two residents, and sometimes to the whole group. At times, it is directed to his own faculty members and partners. A lot could be written on this subject, however, in the final summation, there are only two things to be said. Either you do whatever is necessary to get on the difficult attending's good side, or you respectfully ignore his or her anger but not the person. Of course, the former is better than the latter; however, it takes a lot of energy and thought to stay ethical, moral, respectful, and energized by your work in this sort of situation. The latter tactic takes a certain finesse, but when it works, it can often change the entire situation, and the attending may very well see the error of his or her ways. Always remember that in due time you will be out of that situation, while he or she will remain unchanged.

The Difficult Consultant

The difficult consultant bears mentioning only to warn you and to suggest a way of handling him. The difficult consultant may:

Not be available when you need him
Not come in a timely fashion
Not hit it off with your patient
Not adequately provide the consultation that you
    desire
Not write a report of the consultation immediately
    and legibly
Not call you with a report
Speak to you in a condescending tone
Have a less-experienced doctor do the consultation
    when a more experienced consultant is necessary
Not perform to standards that you have set for yourself

If you are not satisfied with the quality of the consultation, then immediately call a more superior consultant. The next time that you require a consultation, try to have someone else do it.

There is always the option of trying to correct the improper nuances in the consultant by gently telling him how you would prefer things done. This will very often work to your benefit, and both of you will have learned a lesson.

As always, critically evaluate yourself and make sure that you are the kind of consultant that you would like to have called for yourself or your loved ones.

Difficult Hospital Personnel

Hospital personnel include everyone you have contact with inside the hospital, with the exception of the doctors. Very simply, just be nice to them, and they will be nice to you. Show great respect and appreciation for whatever job they do. Remember that most often they are not well paid, have troubles of their own, and that you are just transient; here today, gone tomorrow.

Thank them in any small way that you can. They must have respect for your position, and you must have even more respect for theirs.

If there is a serious problem with any of them, then gently call it to the attention of their superiors, and try to offer a remedial solution. Never verbally attack ancillary personnel.

9

Documentation

Anybody can make history. Only a great man can write it.

—Oscar Wilde

The careful and accurate completion of medical records is not only an important physician responsibility, it is mandatory. Developing good habits of record keeping serves seven essential purposes:

1. Your record is an **aide-memoir** when you next see the patient.
2. A clear, accurate note is a **guide for your colleagues** who may need a quick review when seeing the patient in the years to come for continuity of care.
3. The **clinic summary** should be a concise summation of the many hours of thought, investigation, and consultation that were spent in attempting to unravel the patient's problem.
4. Your notes are records of all diagnostic terms that are required for **case retrieval** in clinical investigations. References to the original pathology reports are essential in all tumor cases.
5. Flawless documentation affords a **justification of payment** by third parties, particularly when significant diagnostic efforts have been made.

6. All medical record notations must be ***timed in compliance*** with medical staff by-laws. Also, always clearly document when an attending physician transfers patient care to another physician.

7. The medical record is a ***legal document*** and may be used in courts of law.

Thus, incomplete or inaccurate records may endanger the patient, inconvenience future clinicians, delay or abrogate payment, relegate the record to oblivion for purposes of research, and serve the courts for any cause.

An accurate record of everything that you do concerning patient care is mandatory for the remainder of your career. This is not only often required by law or statute or local tradition, but primarily and ultimately to provide better patient care. The basic thread throughout this chapter will be to document:

> **Honestly**
> **Completely**
> **Legibly**
> **Timely**

The attending staff and the faculty are ultimately responsible for every act of patient care and documentation that you perform.

It is very important to remember that all documentation, whether handwritten or computer-generated, constitutes a legal article, and can be used in many forums (court, committees, institutions, government agencies) for or against you, and for and against the patient. Remember, if you did not document an event, then it either did not happen, or one could say that it did not occur as you recalled it.

Your signature must be clearly legible. If it is not, then you must print your name beside the signature. You should always write your pager number under your signature.

The use of abbreviations has become prevalent not only in documentation, but also in presentations and casual medical talk. Acronyms can often become confusing, misleading, dangerous, and they are not always universally recognizable. Most institutions have a list of acceptable abbreviations, and the Joint Commission for Accreditation of Hospitals (Appendix A) constantly updates a comprehensive list on their web site.

Patient Charts

History and Physical Examination

The correct format for performing and recording the results of the history and physical examinations is learned in medical school and should be strictly adhered to. The history must be thorough, including not only significant items, but also those seemingly insignificant medical events that may be totally unrelated to the present illness. When documenting the diagnosis or impression, try not to use superlatives or adjectives. For example, "huge ventral hernia," "large wound of the buttocks," "foul smelling sore of the left big toe," etc. Instead, the correct terminology for the diagnosis should be written as "ventral hernia – 10cm × 20cm," "wound of buttocks –24cm × 12cm," "infected wound left big toe." The superlatives and adjectives may be used in the description part of the physical examination.

Be sure to complete all of the blanks. It is impossible to know what organ system may become a problem during the hospitalization, and without a baseline examination, it will be difficult to provide adequate care.

If you are in charge of a particular patient, and a student or a person with less experience has written the history and physical examination, you should first check it in detail and then countersign it. A students' work must always be countersigned immediately.

Progress Notes

Progress notes should be written at least once a day, and more frequently if necessary. A note should be written during each and every visit. Include the date and time of each visit. A helpful, appreciated suggestion is to also print your specialty beside the date and time. Record all salient facts of the visit, as well as any change in the patient's condition, whether good or bad. Write any new or changed laboratory or test values, as well as the results of pathology or x-ray reports. Be very specific and very thorough. Sign your name legibly, and also print it if necessary. Never use a stamp. Always write or record the progress note directly after seeing the patient. Never write a progress note until you have personally seen and examined the patient.

It is a good idea to occasionally tabulate certain events when they are salient. For example, record of a temperature chart of the past few days in a patient with a fever, or hemoglobin levels for the past few days in a patient who may be bleeding. There is nothing wrong with being innovative in the progress notes to help others who are reading the notes and in order to document that you know all of the events that have occurred.

Consultations

1. You Request the Consultation.
Consultations are usually requested of and by more senior residents and fellows, which implies a greater experi-

ence in diagnosis and treatment, and in note writing, which may or may not be true. Consultation requests should be made on a personal basis (i.e., telephone call), as well as a written order. The rules for the request are :

- Write legibly.
- State the precise reason for the consultation.
- State the history as it pertains to the consultation.
- State the results of your physical examination as it pertains to the consultation request.
- State any salient laboratory or diagnostic results.
- If warranted, your request may also provide permission for the consultant to request any tests or perform whatever treatment found to be necessary.
- The request should be communicated directly to the consultant.

2. You are the Consultant
   - Respond as soon as possible.
   - Do not send a more junior consultant than yourself.
   - Familiarize yourself with the patient's chart.
   - Examine the patient without undermining or contesting any diagnosis or treatments that the referring doctor has given.
   - If appropriate, tell the patient what you are thinking, but that his doctor will explain it in detail.

Then, legibly write your diagnosis or impression *and* a detailed explanation. Suggest any changes in the treatment plan, but do not actually write orders for the changes, unless specifically instructed to do so by the referring doctor.

Regardless of what you think, or how you would handle the case, you must immediately speak to the referring doctor regarding your thoughts about the patient's condition and treatment. This task should not be left to a more junior person. Refrain from refuting the referring doctor in writing until you have had a chance to speak with him directly, as very often a "meeting of the minds" will come to an agreed upon plan for the patient's overall benefit.

If additional specialty consultations are necessary, it is the referring doctor who must request them. If appropriate, and if desired by the referring doctor, you should follow the patient with at least daily visits until your services are no longer needed, and you have signed off on the case.

Orders

Writing accurate and legible orders can make the difference between life and death. All orders must be signed with the date and time and your pager number. Be very careful to use only approved abbreviations. For clarity, you should print the name of medications and their dose. Always print the route for the drug to be administered. Any complicated orders should be reviewed in person with the nurse who is in charge of the patient. Any "stat" orders should be directly identified to the nurse, not the ward secretary. Do not leave anything to chance when writing orders. Check and double-check them. *Students may not write orders.*

Operation Reports

1. **Preoperative Note.** The operating surgeon is responsible for a handwritten preoperative note on the day of the operation. This should include:

   1. Diagnosis and short history
   2. Cardiorespiratory status with test results
   3. Laboratory data
   4. Consultations (if applicable)
   5. Special studies (if applicable).
   6. Indications for operation.

7. Surgical procedure proposed.
8. Operation permit consent: *A statement should be included to the effect that the indications for operation, the type of surgical procedure, its implications and possible complications have been discussed with the patient and understood, and that the patient agrees. Also note that the patients' questions were answered.*
9. Medications.
10. Blood available (if applicable).
11. Surgeons: *The names of the attending surgeons should be provided with a statement that the case was discussed, and there was agreement on the plan of action.*
12. Family: *If appropriate, and if the patient desires, family members should be briefed at this point. This discussion should be noted. Note who was present, preferably name and relationship.*
13. Living will/advanced directives: *The chart should be inspected for completeness of these 2 items.*

2. Operative Report. The decision as to who will dictate the operative report should be made by the end of the operation. If you do the major part of the procedure, then you should dictate it; however, some attendings prefer to complete this task themselves.

It must be noted whether the attending surgeon was present for the "key and critical portions of the procedure." This note is important not only for legal reasons but for reimbursement purposes as well.

The dictated operative report has many purposes, all very important. It must be very complete and very accurate. This document will be referred to by other doctors, nurses, billing personnel, insurance companies, regulatory agencies, hospitals, compliance committees, peer-review organizations, lawyers, and your specialty examining board. It is a valuable teaching and research tool. The following is a good format for dictating the Operative Note:

1. Name of person dictating.
2. Name of patient: *essential patient information to properly track the patient.*
3. Date of surgery.
4. Date dictated.
5. Name of surgeon(s).
6. Name of assistant(s).
7. Preoperative diagnosis: *Not to be overstated, reason for performing the surgical procedures.*
8. Postoperative diagnosis: *The pre-diagnosis and post-diagnosis should conform to ICD-9 coding.*
9. Title of operation(s): *A comprehensive and accurate list and description of services provided during the operative setting; each procedure should approximate a known CPT code; note the size of a lesion, the size of the excision, the depth of the excision; note size and precise location of all lacerations individually.*
10. Indications for surgery: *This will aid the billing department and the reviewers.*
11. Type of anesthesia.
12. Description of operation: *In-depth description of the entire operative setting, which must support the diagnoses, the procedural listings, and the indications; it should be noted whether the procedure was more difficult, bilateral, lengthy; indicate all layers of closure; if the wound was not closed, this should be explicitly mentioned; clearly indicate partial or complete excision (hemicolectomy vs. total colectomy); the correct side of the body should be indicated and consistent throughout.*

13. Findings at operation.
14. Complications.
15. Drains and catheters.
16. Estimated blood loss.
17. Total fluid replacement and type.

Do not use superlatives; just be factual. Make it so clear and informative that a doctor reading it 20 years from now will have no questions, nor will a peer reviewer have a problem interpreting it. It is mandatory that you dictate the operative report directly following the procedure.

3. **Postoperative Note.** An "op note" should be written in the progress notes at the end of the operation, so that recovery room staff and floor nurses will know what has been done to their patient prior to receiving the dictated report. This should be simple and complete:

1. Date, service
2. Heading: "OP NOTE"
3. Name of Surgeon
4. Name of Assistant
5. Preoperative Diagnosis
6. Postoperative Diagnosis
7. Operation
8. Anesthesia
9. Findings
10. Complications
11. Drains
12. Estimated blood loss
13. Signature and pager number

Discharge Summary

The discharge summary is usually dictated, but can be handwritten. This important record must not be delegated to medical students or members of the medical team who are not familiar with the case. The format is as follows:

1. Date of admission
2. Date of discharge
3. Chief complaint
4. History of present illness
5. Hospital course
6. Procedures performed with dates
7. Laboratory tests done and results (only when directly related to diagnosis)
8. Special tests (only when related to diagnosis)
9. X-ray and pathology descriptions
10. Medications
11. Blood received
12. Daily trends in temperature, blood pressure, etc.
13. Complications of hospitalization
14. Discharge condition
15. Discharge disposition
16. Discharge medications, diet, activities
17. Follow-up (very specific, i.e., who, when, where)
18. Final diagnosis (list all of them)
19. Signature

Face Sheet

The face sheet of the patient's chart is very important to the hospital for billing and outcome reporting purposes. Usually, the hospital will complete the form. When it is your job, then just fill in the blanks.

Informed Consent

Informed consent is the legal and ethical right that a patient has to be fully informed about his condition and treatments, so that the patient can participate in all the phases and choices concerning his or her health care. The physician has an ethical and a legal duty to inform the patient in language that the patient can understand, so that the patient can decide what is best.

A complete informed consent must include the following elements:

- The nature of the treatment or procedure
- Reasonable alternatives to the proposed treatment
- The relevant risks, benefits, and uncertainties relating to each alternative
- Assessment of the patient understanding
- The acceptance of the treatment by the patient

Many books have been written on informed consent, and controversy will shroud the concept for a long time to come. However, the interns and residents must become experts on this subject by the first time they find themselves before the patient or his family in a situation of explaining and requesting informed consent.

It will be obvious to you that neither two situations will be the same, nor will any two informed consents be the same. However, in every situation, you must adhere to the basic concepts, which are:

- Nature and seriousness of the treatment or procedure
- Alternatives to the treatment or procedure
- Risks, benefits, and uncertainties of the treatment or procedure

When special circumstances arise, there are special remedies for them, but the correct protocol must be observed. When in doubt, call upon the nursing supervisor or your attending for help.

DNR

Do not resuscitate orders appear to throw a cloud over a patient's chart. Similar to other medical decisions, the decision to attempt to retrieve the life of a patient who suffers cardiopulmonary arrest involves a very careful consideration of the potential likelihood for clinical benefit, taking into account the patient's general physical condition, his prognosis, and his preferences for the intervention and its likely outcome.

I will not delve into all of the nuances and examples of DNR and CPR. Most institutions have policies about this subject, and usually well-written protocols. You should become very familiar with them very early on in your training.

Living Will

In 1991, the Federal government enacted the *Patient Self-Determination Act*, requiring that patients be informed about their right to participate in health-care decisions, including their right to have an advance directive. Advance directives are broken down into two broad categories: instructive and proxy. The *Living Will* is one type of instructive directive; however, there are others such as no transfusion and no CPR. The proxy directive is generally a *Durable Power of Attorney for Health Care*, which permits the designation of a surrogate medical decision-maker of the patient's choosing. This surrogate is empowered to make all medical decisions for the patient, in the event he or she is incapacitated.

All hospitals ask each patient whether they have a living will. If not, they are given the opportunity to have one on the spot.

You should be familiar with your patient's living will. If a surrogate has been appointed, and your patient is incapacitated, then you must treat the surrogate as though he was the patient, for matters of informed consent.

Prescriptions

Use the standard hospital prescription form. Fill it out completely and legibly. It is good practice to print the entire prescription so that no error in interpretation are possible. Following your signature, print your name and pager number (with area code). Make sure that you circle the maximum number of pills to be prescribed, as well as the refill/no refill space.

Always record the prescription as well as any refills in the patient's chart. Be very careful to whom you give the prescription. Be vigilant with those patients requesting refills for narcotics or mood-changing medications.

Letters, Authorizations, Status Reports

You will frequently be called upon to write letters for patients. If the request is legitimate, you should graciously do it. If you determine that it is nonsense, then just tell the patient that you are unable to comply with his request.

Authorizations for durable medical equipment often require a letter from you. This should be done quickly, as the patient is most likely in immediate need.

Insurance companies, home health agencies, and governmental agencies, for instance, frequently request status reports and forms on patients. This is usually presented to you by means of a standard form for you to fill in the blanks. These forms should be completed with the patient's chart in front of you. Be honest and complete.

A last word about your written notes. If you need to correct something in any written medical document at a later point, under no circumstance should you erase it, black it out, scratch it out, or white it out. Place one line through it, so that it can still be read, place the date and your initials adjacent to it, and write a new note, or an addendum at the bottom. Do not write the new note in the margins or between lines.

10

Presentations

You don't have to be a chicken to make an omelet.

—MARK TWAIN

Don't let it end like this. Tell them I said something.

—Last Words of Pancho Villa

You will often be called upon to make presentations, sometimes to small groups and not infrequently to large and austere groups. It behooves you to use the small group presentations to perfect and streamline your technique in preparation and delivery so that your large and/or important group presentations will be very professional. Formal presentations are an art form. A really good one is as enjoyable to present as it is to observe. Once you make the presentation, store it away for the next time. The following are suggestions to facilitate your preparation and presentation.

Preparation of Slides

1. Use Power Point.
2. Do not be too concerned with slide backgrounds, intricate title slides, animations or fancy graphics; they can distract from your presentation.

3. Use only one font. No fancy fonts.
4. No light print like yellow or pink.
5. Use footnotes. Give credit where credit is due.
6. Try to integrate into your presentation, and give credit to any work done by your attendings, the department, and/or the institution.
7. Graphs must be uncomplicated, but detailed enough for the audience to quickly interpret them.
8. Charts should not have a lot of barely readable numbers, but should be reduced to their essence.
9. Adjust the complexity and the language of the presentation to the audience, i.e., students, residents, attendings, nurses, lay public, etc.
10. You and a friend should review the entire presentation, double-checking the spelling and order of the slides.
11. Keep in mind that slides are only an adjunct to your presentation. You are the focus of attention.

Presentation

1. Arrive early.
2. Order needed equipment in advance, and make sure it works. Make sure you know how to operate it.
3. Try using some sort of "memory stick" rather than a CD. It is a lot cooler! It is always a good idea to have a backup disk with you.
4. Dress for the occasion. It shows, and demands respect.
5. Stand up, regardless of how many presentations you have seen where the presenter is seated.
6. Do not lean against anything.
7. Keep your hands out of your pockets.
8. Use a laser pointer if available.

9. Look at your audience. Do not ever look at the floor, or the ceiling. This gives the body language of lying.

10. Do not rub your chin or cover your mouth with your hand.

11. Only look at the screen for brief intervals.

12. Do not read from the slides. Your audience will be reading them. It is disconcerting to repeat what they are reading.

13. Do not cross your arm in front of your body when pointing to the screen. Use your hand closest to the screen.

14. Never apologize for a bad slide. If the slide is bad, do not use it.

15. A certain amount of humor is permitted as long as it is in context.

16. Ask for questions or comments. Be prepared to answer.

17. At the end, simply say "thank you."

The Mortality and Morbidity Conference

Tell me and I forget.
Show me and I remember
Teach me and I learn.

—BENJAMIN FRANKLIN

The Mortality and Morbidity Conference (M & M) is certainly the most important hour of the week for residents and their teachers. Here is the last bastion of medical intellect, competition, showmanship, and debate. And, the most important component in the M & M is the absolutely perfect presentation, which requires extensive preparation.

Preparation

1. Collect all of the facts of the case. If certain historical information is not readily available, search it out.
   If necessary, call previous doctors, clinics, hospitals, and if appropriate, the patient's family. The data, regardless of how trivial, must be sought.

2. Discuss the case to be presented with your attending. This is not only a matter of courtesy, it may also give you additional, detailed information, and it will also prevent you from getting blind-sided by questions from that attending. If the attending for that case cannot be present for the conference, the case should not be presented.

3. Only residents who thoroughly know the case, the main issues, and the controversies surrounding the complication, should be presenting. Thus, the case should be presented by the most senior resident who will conduct himself as if he were the attending surgeon and the patient was from his private office.

Presentation

Each institution's M & M Conference has its little idio-syncrasies not limited to specific seating arrangements, attendance, and the precise way in which the case is presented. While some (very few) places do not take the conference very seriously, you have the opportunity to elevate it to a new level by preparing your presentation in the following format.

1. Prepare a brief, **printed summary** to serve as a sort of "database." Do not waste time reviewing facts. Members of the audience will have more time to formulate their thoughts and questions. Include line drawings if applicable.

2. Have **audiovisual aids** available (overhead projector, slide projector, microscope projector, etc.). A picture is worth a thousand words, and it certainly makes your discussion more objective.

3. **Dress** for the occasion. Carry yourself as though you were the professor. Review the chapter on "Presentations."

4. Even though the surgical operation is probably the central event, it is not the most important event. Present a very clear, specific, and anatomically precise description of the **technical operation and the findings at the time of surgery.**

5. Attempt to anticipate the **questions** you might be asked, and incorporate the answers into your presentation.

6. **Avoid the use of terms** like "extremely difficult," "massive," "odd looking," "weird," "never seen that before." This is not the time for subjectivity. What is exaggerated for some may be commonplace for others.

7. Review **x-rays** with the radiologist, and better yet, have the radiologist attend the conference. Never tell the audience that you could not get the x-rays.

8. Do not waste the audience's time telling them of **laboratory values**. Write them on the blackboard, or better, include them in a printed handout at the beginning of the presentation.

9. The M & M should be fun (we surgeons are a morbid bunch). The dynamic of the meeting is the interplay between the knowledge and the ignorance of both the residents and the audience. Inappropriate questions as well as inappropriate answers determine who walks out with their heads held high. Therefore, **rehearse your presentation** with your fellow residents and/or your attending.

10. Following your immaculate presentation, there will be a dedicated time for **questions**.

a. Be polite. Show respect to the questioner, even if the question is dumb and shows a complete lack of understanding of the case.

b. You may say "I do not know." If you believe that somebody else in the room knows the answer, you may ask them to respond, but do not put them on the spot if the answer is going to be another "I do not know."

c. If you are well prepared and your presentation is complete, the questions will be directed at your thought process rather than the details of the case.

11. Put the **case in context** with the known and generally accepted practice of the art of surgery. Cite references from recognized and not-so-recognized authorities on the subject, both for and against the evaluation and treatment of the patient in question. The literature you cite may be an ally or an enemy. It should be presented in a balanced format.

12. The **summary of the case** and its complications should be short, honest, and sometimes humbling. This is where an admission of guilt is made if necessary. It is in this closing statement where those in the room will or will not see the fruits of their labors in helping to create a mature surgeon.

13. Finally, the **attending** should respectfully be called upon for comment. Most likely, she has been quite vocal throughout, but she should have a dedicated moment to have the last word.

The purpose of the M & M conference is to teach and learn. The proceedings are protected from disclosure in court, and therefore unabashed honesty is demanded and expected. There should be no attempt to cover-up or to protect anybody.

This has been only a brief description and a few suggestions to make your presentation at the M & M Conference more effective. There are books on the entire subject. We suggest reading *Gordon's Guide to the Surgical Morbidity and Mortality Conference.*[1]

---

[1] Gordon, Leo A., Hanley & Belfus Medical Publishers, 1995.

12

The 80-Hour Week

Sometimes it is not enough to do our best; we must do what is required.

—SIR WINSTON CHURCHILL

The educational goals of residency training programs and the learning objectives of residents must not be compromised by excessive clinical service obligations. The Accreditation Council on Graduate Medical Education (ACGME) has charged sponsoring institutions with ensuring that formal written policies governing resident duty hours be established at both the institutional and program level.

Each sponsored program must have a formal written policy on resident duty hours. The ACGME regulations are listed below. It should be understood that each program and institution has adapted these rules; however, the minimum requirements apply to all.

- Duty hours must not exceed 80 hours per week, averaged over 4 weeks. Duty hours are defined as:
  - All clinical activities relating to the residency program
  - All academic activities relating to the residency program
  - All administrative duties relating to the residency program

- All patient care duties
- All conferences
- All on call time
- Residents must be given 10 hours off for rest and personal activities between duty periods and after call.
- In-house call must occur no more frequently than every third night, averaged over four weeks.
- Resident assignments must not exceed 24 hours maximum, continuous on-site duty, with up to 6 additional hours permitted for patient transfer and other activities defined in RRC requirements.
- A resident must not be assigned new patients after 24 hours of continuous duty.
- Resident time spent in the hospital during at-home call must be counted towards the 80 hours. At-home call is not subject to the every third night limitation.
- "Moonlighting." (spare time work)
  - Must be approved by the program director. Some programs specifically forbid it.
  - Must not interfere with your ability to achieve the goals and objectives of the educational program.
  - Must be monitored to ensure you comply with the program and institutional policies.
  - Work outside the residency program and the institution does not count against the 80 hours.
  - Internal moonlighting (i.e., within the program or institution) must be counted toward the 80 hour weekly limit on duty hours.
- All residents must be provided with one day in seven days, free from all educational and clinical responsibilities, averaged over a 4-week period, inclusive of call. "One day" is defined as one continuous 24-hour period.

- Duty hours must be monitored by the program. Most programs will require weekly written reports and a quarterly time study. Some programs satisfy the reporting requirements online.
- Program directors must develop and have in place policies to prevent and counteract the effects of resident fatigue.
- Back-up support must be provided when needed.

Always consult the rules specific to your residency training program and hospital. These rules must be taken very seriously because your program could lose its accreditation if they are violated. Some states have statutes concerning these rules, thereby making them the law. If broken, someone could actually be fined or go to jail.

13

The Boards

Perhaps the most valuable result of all education is the ability to make yourself do the thing you have to do, when it ought to be done, whether you like it or not; it is the first lesson that ought to be learned; and however early a man's training begins, it is probably the last lesson that he learns thoroughly.

—THOMAS H. HUXLEY (1825-1895)

Preparation for eventual board certification begins the day you start your training, regardless of specialty. All boards are composed of three parts: a written examination, an oral examination, and some kind of case log. The written exam is fairly straightforward. Throughout your training and after, you will systematically study all of the disciplines, and take a multiple choice test. If you pass, you will be permitted to take the oral exam, which will not only test your knowledge, but will actually test your personal skills by demonstrating to the examiner(s) that you are the kind of person who will be safe enough to be considered board certified.

The Operative Record

The maintenance and reporting of the resident operative record is an integral part of your educational experience, and the accreditation of the residency program depends on how you fulfill the responsibility. Each resident must record each operation performed or assisted, in an ongoing fashion, thereby preparing an operative log of his own case experience. The American Board of Surgery Residency Review Committee (RRC) has its own web site, as do most of the specialty surgery boards, so that the operative log can be directly entered online in a contemporaneous fashion. The various Boards have their own format and requirements for entering data, and usually request CPT codes along with the operative report. This data must be kept up-to-date as it provides the backbone of the Residency program's accreditation, as well as your application for certification by the board.

The In-Service Exam

Most specialties including General Surgery offer an in-service examination. This provides the program director an opportunity for an annual evaluation of the core curriculum. Your performance will be compared to that of all other residents in your specialty in your year of training. This record will become a part of your permanent resident file and could be a deciding factor in determining whether you advance to the senior year, as well as whether you graduate. The examination scores may be included in any letter of recommendation/support for future employment, as well as for sitting for the boards.

You can see that constant preparation is necessary. If your training program has a course of study for the exam, do not miss a single session. If it does not, you should organize your colleagues and systematically tackle every discipline, the so-called core curriculum that will be on the exam. Constantly review the basic sciences. Keep yourself up-to-date on current readings.

Read everything you can put your hands on. Study for this examination as you will eventually study for the Boards. It is your job.

Tips for Remembering and Studying for Tests

It goes without saying that you already know how to study. After all, you graduated medical school, and that was no easy task. Nonetheless, read these tips on studying and perhaps you will gain some new ideas.

- It is important to form strong impressions of things you wish to remember with as much detail as possible, but separate the wheat from the chaff.
- Study with the intention of remembering by mentally repeating or by writing the item.
- Try to do something as soon as possible with the information you have learned.
- Try to associate a new fact with something that you already know.
- Review what you have learned previously, a few days after you reviewed the material for the first time.
- Try to learn material as a whole instead of isolated, separate parts so that it fits into context.
- When studying one subject and switching to another, take a brief rest. When changing subjects, try to go after the break to a topic that is entirely different.
- Have confidence in your memory and your ability to retain information.
- Do not skip classes or assigned reading material.
- Stay awake. Sit in front of the room. What ever it takes, be aware and stay focused.
- Stay focused on the topic. Do not let your mind wonder by daydreaming about another subject.

- Realize that success on a test is similar to the success in patient care. Both will give you pleasure.
- When studying, it may be necessary to read aloud to keep on the subject.
- Know definitions. Do not use terms unless you understand and know the definition of the terminology.
- Stay alert. Turn off your telephone. Turn off your TV. CONCENTRATE.

14

The Interview

Sow a thought and you reap an action;
Sow an act and you reap a habit;
Sow a habit and you reap a character;
Sow a character and you reap a destiny.

—BUDDHIST PROVERB

Placement for training positions in surgery and the surgical subspecialties has historically been highly competitive. Today, obtaining one of these sacred residencies or fellowships is more of a challenge, considering their decreasing numbers, the increasing quality and credentials of the applicants, and, in most instances, the rather mechanical "match." From start to finish of this grueling, complicated, meticulous, and often expensive process the student (or resident) is required to portray his or her life in the best possible light, so as to impress the reviewer(s) to the point where he or she will get the job. So many factors in this selection process are, in reality, so completely out of your control that you had at least better increase your chances of acceptance by making an immaculate application and interview.

The essence of this chapter is provided by experienced reviewers who have read thousands of applications, have interviewed hundreds of applicants, and who have accepted only a few candidates. These are only a few tips.

The Preparation

You began to prepare when you entered medical school:

- You made good grades.
- You tried for honors courses.
- You volunteered for anything and everything.
- You sat in front of the lecture room.
- You worked in a research laboratory.
- You asked good questions.
- You read this book and lived the spirit of it.

During the clinical years:

- You arrived earlier and left later than your fellow students.
- You worked hard to learn and secondarily to impress your attendings and residents.
- You asked good questions.
- You listened carefully.
- You continued to work in the research laboratory.
- You worked towards getting your name listed on publications.
- You nurtured your relationship with the professor in-charge of your research laboratory. Hopefully he or she is going to write a letter of recommendation for you.
- You did not antagonize any secretaries in the department. They are really important. Secretaries "run the world."
- The residents and fellows you rotated with have sterling comments to make about your work. When questioned by an attending, an angry resident can do you a great deal of harm, or good.
- You read this book, and lived the spirit of it.

If you are applying for a residency or fellowship position from a residency or a fellowship position, then your mission becomes more detailed and more competitive.

- Applicants named in several publications look great.
- Applicants with transferable research grants are irresistible.
- You must read this book again and live by the spirit of it.

The Application

The written application is the easiest part of your documentation. Just do it correctly, neatly, and timely. It is at this time, that you might communicate with the secretaries or coordinators of the institutions that you are applying to. Be absolutely professional, courteous, and just plain nice. They often have a "say". You can be sure that if you antagonize one of them, or in frustration, speak harshly to one of them, it will get back to the chairman, and you will not get the job.

- Type the entire application.
- Do not use initials anywhere on the application.
- Do not be too trite or clichéd in your personal statement.
- Attempt to record your greatest achievements in a moderate fashion. In other words, the reviewers can also read between the lines.

The Interview

A discussion of this aspect of the application process is the main purpose of this chapter. The interview is your time to come out, to shine, to impress, and perhaps to beg a little. Everything must be perfect. However, being perfect is usually not enough. You must be better than all of the other applicants. Your history speaks for itself and is unalterable. Now you have to show the real you.

- Be early for your interview.
- Do you know how to dress?

For men, dark suit (no pinstripes), subdued but sharp necktie, polished shoes, hair well cut and groomed. No jewelry except for a wedding band (if you are married). Facial hair in some programs is frowned upon.

For women, dark pants suit or dress suit, minimal jewelry, only one small earring in each ear, no high heels, above all, dress conservatively (certain interviewers resent that an applicant may believe that showing a little cleavage or thigh might influence their decision.) Actually, it may negatively influence it.

- Often, secretaries, coordinators, interns and residents will be around to assist in the interview process. Get close to them. Talk to them. Be nice to them. They will be asked for their opinion about you.
- Shake hands solidly, not like a wet fish.
- Do not fidget.
- Sit up straight on the edge of your chair.
- Address each interviewer by his or her name. Never look at the ceiling, the floor, the table, or into space. Make eye contact.
- <u>Never</u> say "yeh." Always say "yes sir, no sir (or mam)." Never say, "you know?" Do not say "I probably..." Say "I definitely..." or "I immediately..." Sound like you mean it.
- Answer all questions without beating around the bush. Be direct, forceful, assertive, and certain. Make sure that you answer questions in the context that they are asked.
- Smile.

- Do not embellish too much. Certainly do not brag.
- The idea is to get the interviewer to like you and trust you. All of the details of your life are on the written application. The interview makes it all personal, and helps fill in the spaces between the words.
- Demonstrate your compassion and your ability to work hard.
- Make the interviewer eager to be with you for the next few years. He will be able to tell in a few minutes that you are the kind of person who will be a pleasure to teach.
- Read this book again.

The Match

Many candidates for residency and fellowship positions will be applying through the "match," the details of which are beyond the scope of this book. The match is a sort of computer game, which at a point in the process, takes out the humanism and relegates your future to a computer program. Actually, it is most likely, the fairest way to deal with so many applications.

Do not violate any of the match rules or dates.

Medical – Legal

Becoming involved in a law suit is like being ground to bits in a slow mill; it's being roasted at a slow fire; it's being stung to death by a single bee; it's being drowned by drops; it's going mad by grains. Hundreds of thousands of people are exposed to such torture each year, some of them actually choosing to initiate the process. They invariably find the experience painful, protracted and expensive. When it has run its course, they often realize that it was futile. Yet there remains a queue of victims impatient for their turn.

—CHARLES DICKENS

Malpractice

Malpractice is defined as "treatment which is contrary to accepted medical standards and which produces injurious results in patients." Since most medical malpractice actions are based on laws governing negligence, the law recognizes that medicine is an inexact art and that there can be no absolute liability. Thus, the cause of action is usually "failure" of the defendant and/or physician to exercise that reasonable degree of skill, learning, care, and treatment ordinarily possessed by others of the same profession in the community.

Not only is the definition confusing and open-ended to the average physician, the entire process can become unnerving for not only the physician, but also for the purported victim as well. For many reasons, it will make your life much easier if you can avoid the malpractice system. To keep yourself out of trouble, you must practice medicine as though trouble were right around the corner, virtually for the rest of your life. Briefly, here are some rough guidelines to live by in order to stay out of the courtroom:

- Do not practice medicine beyond the scope of your abilities and level of training.
- Write notes clearly, legibly, and contemporaneously. Include your signature, the date, and time.
- Be thorough, noting positive and negative findings.
- Record in the chart every patient visit and family member discussion.
- Double check your written orders.
- Fill in all of the blanks on forms.
- Use only recognized abbreviations (Appendix B).
- Obtain adequate informed consent.
- Never, ever, alter medical records. Corrections can be made as a separate entry, signed and dated. Never write between the lines or in the margins.
- All written and called-in prescriptions must be entered in to the patient's chart.
- All telephone calls from or about a patient should be noted in the patient's chart.
- Respond quickly to patients' concerns and telephone calls.
- Always be available.
- Remember HIPAA
- Be honest. Be compassionate.

Legal Documents

Just about everything that you write or type into a computer during your training could be considered a legal document and, therefore, could be admissible in court. The patient's medical record is certainly a legal document, and requires great care and forethought when written. Once entered into the chart, it cannot be removed or altered, except by very explicit means. And even those means still leave the original writings intact and visible.

Responding to a Subpoena or Requests from Attorneys

If you should receive a subpoena to produce documents, or any other request for a medical record, you must immediately and personally give it to the legal affairs department of the hospital. Note in your little black book the date and time and who it was handed to. Under no circumstance should you neglect it, delay it, or respond yourself. The failure to timely comply with a subpoena could place you in contempt of court, with subsequent fine and/or imprisonment.

A request from an attorney for information about a patient must also be immediately given to the legal department for disposition. You are also required to give a copy of the letter to the chairman of your department. Do not give it to anyone else. Do not talk to anyone about it. This is very important. Keep your mouth shut. These letters often appear quite benign, but could be the beginning of a lot of grief for you.

Testifying

It is very possible that you will be called to testify as a witness in a deposition or trial about a patient who you somehow came in contact with. The legal department will help you with this. Unfortunately, this is a necessary, unwanted part of your education. The only thing you have to do is be honest, knowledgeable, believable and compassionate.

There is not enough room in this book to give the subject of testifying any justice. However, you can prepare yourself for the inevitable time when you will be called upon to testify for either the prosecution, the defense, or for yourself. When that time arrives, your attorney will prepare you for the occasion. The purpose here is to encourage you to begin thinking towards that fateful time and to return to this section occasionally to reinforce the way you should behave in a court of law. These suggestions and observations could help you one day.

- Few things will cause you more anger, frustration, and anxiety than dealing with an attorney.
- Keep your "cool" when dealing with attorneys.
- Jurors do not like hotheads or smart alecks.
- Always be the nicest person in the room. Judges and jurors like pleasant witnesses.
- A good witness is a teacher.
- Study your testimony and chart as you would for your most important final exam.
- Never promise a result to a patient. The promise may be repeated to you in court.
- Do not try to impress the attorneys or jury with your importance.
- Dress for court as you would for an important interview. Look clean, pressed, and professional. Shine your shoes. No fancy watches or jewelry.
- Make eye contact with the attorneys, judge, and jury.
- It is better to say "I do not know." No lying. No wavering.
- Do not fidget. Keep your hands off your face. Never look at the floor or ceiling.
- For video testimony, look at the camera when speaking.

- Use plain English. Avoid medical terminology or abbreviations that the jury will not understand.
- Watch out for convoluted or compound questions.
- Do not carry a medical textbook into court or to a deposition. Anything in the book can be used, negatively.
- If an attorney quotes your prior depositions or some medical literature, you have the right to see the entire text. Beware of statements taken out of context.
- Answer to the lawyer; explain to the jury.
- Juries love pictures and diagrams. Use them liberally. Ask the judge if you can step down from the stand to explain or demonstrate a point. Juries like that also.
- When asked to respond to a hypothetical question, be absolutely sure it fits the facts of the case.
- Do not use language (terminology) unless you know the definition. You can count on the attorney asking you to define terms such as "sensitivity" or "specificity."
- If you attribute a disease or injury to a cause, be sure you are correct, and it is supported by the peer-reviewed literature.
- Know the facts of every case you are involved in. Someday you may have to explain the diagnosis and treatment to a group of non-medical strangers (a jury).
- For the purpose of testimony, symptoms do not equal a diagnosis.
- Be sure you know the patient's chart in great detail before any testimony. Read your notes.
- Be sure you know the literature on the topic before you give testimony.

- Ask the attorney to explain the legal facts of the case to you. If you do not understand, ask him again.
- If you are presented with a summons stating that you are party to a lawsuit, keep your mouth shut. Discuss it only with your chairman and the legal department. There is one exception to this rule: You may discuss it with your personal attorney. If you find it necessary to retain a personal attorney, he or she should be a litigator who is very familiar with medical malpractice.
- Never fail to disclose on any employment application that you were named in a case, even if the case was dropped. Read the application questions carefully, and answer honestly. If you have survived a lawsuit, have an attorney help you draw up a letter of explanation of what happened. Keep this letter forever; you will have to use it to explain disclosure in future employment applications.

Conflict of Interest

During your training, there will be opportunities to accept gifts from vendors, patients, students, etc. The rules pertaining to this vary among institutions. The laws of some states and the Federal laws are quite specific and should be researched. As a rule of thumb, do not accept anything from anybody in exchange for favors or for the use of a product. That should keep you out of trouble.

Child Abuse

Child abuse takes many forms, including child sexual abuse, pedophilia, physical abuse, neglect, emotional neglect, failure to thrive, and Munchausen by proxy syndrome. Interns and residents, and physicians in general, are in a position daily to discern these travesties on children. Most states mandate that physicians must, by law, report to the authorities these aberrant acts. The possibility of child abuse must be constantly in the back of your mind. If you suspect you have seen the results of such an act, you should either consult a nursing supervisor before telephoning the police, or just call the police. The law will protect any person who reports child abuse, so long as the report is not made with malice of intent.

The laws are less specific for elder abuse; however, it should always be a question in your mind when treating debilitated older patients.

16

HIPAA

The de-identification of protected health information has turned presentations on bedside rounds into masterpieces of obfuscation. Not the name, nor the initials, and not even the exact age of the patient may be used. This sad state of affairs now confronts all clinical research in the USA.

—SUSAN GALANDIUK, M.D.
(*British Journal of Surgery* 2004; 91: 259-261)

The *Health Insurance Portability and Accountability Act of 1996 (HIPAA)* was instituted in the US to ensure the protection of individuals' health information, while also allowing communication between parties involved with patient care. It was not until 1999, however, when the US Department of Health and Human Services developed the Privacy Rule that made implementation of HIPAA mandatory. Effective April 2003, organizations (i.e., "covered entities") subject to HIPAA regulations are required to comply with patient information protection policies. "Covered entities" refer to health plans, healthcare providers, and health care clearinghouses.

Required disclosures of identifiable individual health information include a request by a patient for his/her information, or a request by the US Department of Health and Human Services in special instances, such as a review. The privacy rule outlines six permitted disclosures of individual health information, including the following:

1. Per request of the patient
2. For treatment, payment, and healthcare operations
3. To individuals identified by the patient, who may be informed; in emergency situations, the healthcare provider must use his/her professional judgment to determine the best interest of the patient
4. Incidental disclosure
5. Limited data set with the removal of certain individual identifiers
6. Public interest, which encompasses disclosures required by law; public health activities; abuse, neglect, and domestic violence; health oversight activities; judicial and administrative proceedings; law enforcement purposes; decedents; cadaver organ and tissue donation; research with permission of governing body, such as Institutional Review Board; threat to health or society; essential government functions; and workers compensation

State governments reserve the right to have supplemental policies to further increase patient privacy protection. Check with your institution to determine additional policies and guidelines.

In short, treat identifiable health information as patient property. Be careful how, where, and to whom you discuss and distribute patient information. Protection of patient privacy rights is required by law.

Suggestions for HIPAA Compliance

- Be aware of your surroundings. Do not discuss patients in public places such as elevators, waiting rooms, public hallways, and lobbies.
- Dispose of identifiable health information, such as patient lists, in the appropriate manner. Most

hospitals have labeled containers for material that is to be shredded.
- Do not publicly display patient information . This includes both in hospitals and outpatient clinics (i.e., do not leave patients charts unattended).
- When discussing scenarios or presenting a case to individuals not directly involved in the care of a patient, do not disclose identifiable patient information.
- Do not identify patients over the internet.

HIPAA at a Glance

What Is HIPAA?

- Governs the use and disclosure of protected health information (PHI) that is created or received by a covered entity that relates to:
  - The physical or mental health of an individual (living or deceased)
  - The provision of health care
  - The payment for health care
  - Identifies the individual or reasonably may be used to identify the individual
- Gives individuals the following rights:
- The right to...
  - Request restrictions on use or disclosure of their personal health information
  - Access medical records (including research records)
  - Amend medical records
  - An accounting of disclosure of their personal health information
  - Request alternate confidential communications
  - Lodge complaint with covered entity and/or the Department for Health and Human Services

- Administrative requirements. The covered entity must—
  - Designate a privacy official
  - Develop policies and procedures that are HIPAA compliant
  - Provide privacy training to the workforce
  - Implement administrative, technical, and physical safeguards to protect the privacy of personal health information
  - Develop sanctions for violations of the HIPAA Privacy Rule
  - Meet the documentation requirements
- Enforcement/penalties (individual, not institutional)
  - Civil penalties
    - $100 for each violation, up to $25,000/person/year.
    - Liability exists if a person knew, or reasonably should have known, of a violation and did not try to rectify the situation.
  - Criminal penalties
    - Knowing: Up to $50,000/year and/or imprisonment of up to 1 year
    - False pretenses: Up to $100,000/year and/or imprisonment of up to 5 years
    - Intent to sell, transfer, or use for commercial advantage, personal gain or malicious harm: Up to $250,000/year and/or imprisonment of up to 10 years
- Impact on researchers
  - Recruitment of subjects.
  - If a subject refuses to authorize the use and disclosure of public health information, the individual cannot participate in the research study.

   ○ Accounting for disclosures.
      ✓ Preparatory to research
      ✓ Waiver of authorization
      ✓ Decedent data
- Allowable uses and disclosures of PHI for research.
   ○ Authorization from subject
   ○ Waiver of authorization from IRB
   ○ Use of de-identified data
   ○ Use of limited data set
   ○ Preparatory to research
   ○ Decedent data

It is obvious that HIPAA has necessitated a whole new nomenclature for physicians, all individuals in the health care industry, and certainly for the patients who are protected by it. Interestingly, HIPAA is nothing new to physicians. In 400 BC, E. Hippocrates, acclaimed as the father of medicine, proclaimed in his oath that we should uphold the privacy of our patients. This is also addressed in the modern version of the *Hippocratic Oath*.

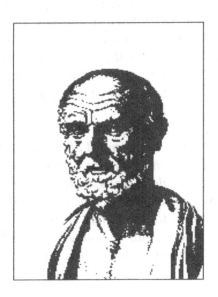

Hippocratic Oath—Classic Version

I swear by Apollo Physician and Asclepius and Hygieia and Panaceia and all the gods and goddesses, making them my witnesses, that I will fulfill according to my ability and judgment this oath and this covenant:

To hold him who has taught me this art as equal to my parents and to live my life in partnership with him, and if he is in need of money to give him a share of mine, and to regard his offspring as equal to my brothers in male lineage and to teach them this art—if they desire to learn i—without fee and covenant; to give a share of precepts and oral instruction and all the other learning to my sons and to the sons of him who has instructed me and to pupils who have signed the covenant and have taken an oath according to the medical law, but no one else.

I will apply dietetic measures for the benefit of the sick according to my ability and judgment; I will keep them from harm and injustice.

I will neither give a deadly drug to anybody who asked for it, nor will I make a suggestion to this effect. Similarly I will not give to a woman an abortive remedy. In purity and holiness I will guard my life and my art.

I will not use the knife, not even on sufferers from stone, but will withdraw in favor of such men as are engaged in this work.

Whatever houses I may visit, I will come for the benefit of the sick, remaining free of all intentional injustice, of all mischief and in particular of sexual relations with both female and male persons, be they free or slaves.

What I may see or hear in the course of the treatment or even outside of the treatment in regard to the life of men, which on no account one must spread abroad, I will keep to myself, holding such things shameful to be spoken about.

If I fulfill this oath and do not violate it, may it be granted to me to enjoy life and art, being honored with fame among all men for all time to come; if I transgress it and swear falsely, may the opposite of all this be my lot.

Assorted Affairs

On Call

On Call in the Hospital

On call duty in the hospital can be one of those necessary evils, if you permit it to be. Being that it is necessary, why not make the very most of the occasion. This time spent away from family, friends, and your own bed, gives you several opportunities:

1. A time to study.
2. An opportunity to learn in real emergency situations, without the convenience and relative safety of attending staff and numerous residents.
3. An opportunity to do more difficult cases, because fewer senior residents will be on call with you.
4. An opportunity to learn when tired. This will condition you for the rest of your life.

Complaining about being on call serves no useful purpose. Just take it on the chin and go about your business. Learn to love it. This is what you signed up for, so do not dread it—embrace it!

Research

> *Research is what I'm doing when I don't know what I'm doing.*
>
> —Werner Von Braun

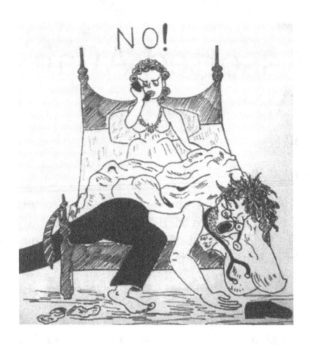

Medical doctors are physicians first, and scientists second. The advanced state of modern medicine has been made possible only by the hard work of our ever inquisitive forefathers. It is our turn to carry on this very important and ancient tradition of intellectual curiosity, discovery, and inventiveness in medicine. There is no place for complacency in medical thought. It is necessary to keep one's eyes, ears, and mind open to the never-ending river of questions generated by today's practice of the healing arts.

Ideas for research are limited only by one's imagination and perseverance, and this provides the nidus for tomorrow's advancements in every aspect of the practice of medicine. Always be on the lookout for questions that need answers, for disease processes that beg for elucidation and treatment, for instruments that need an operation (or vice versa), and for better and newer ways of doing things.

Do not be hesitant to discuss ideas with your attendings, your colleagues, or the appropriate laboratory people. Jot down your ideas in your little black book so that they are not forgotten. Remember, no idea is too insignificant.

Many general surgery residencies require one year of research. If you are considering a career in academic medicine, research and publishing will be mandatory. If you are a student anticipating a career in surgery, now is the time to get involved with one of the many research activities taking place in your medical school. Interviewers at residency training programs are very impressed with students who have participated in research projects. The same goes for those seeking fellowship positions. Regardless of what stage of your training, get involved. It is not only personally very rewarding, but also, in some little, or large way, it serves the cause for the advancement of medicine.

Most universities web sites list the ongoing research projects by department.

History

The history of medicine has been well documented for centuries. We learn from those who came before us as well as those who are in our midst. These inquisitive and inventive minds have shaped our profession into what it is today, to say nothing of the countless sick and injured people whom they have helped through the millennia. Many of the illnesses, procedures, and instruments that we use still bear their names, so it is important for us to know who they were, and are, what they did to enrich our specialty, and why they did it.

'Do not pass up a name without performing at least a cursory search for the individual. Do not pass up the history section of the books that you will read about medicine and surgery. Do not be timid about using the names of the great men and women who have made medicine what it is today.

We truly do stand on the shoulders of giants.

Left Handedness

Society is not sympathetic to the left-handed persons. Surgery is a right-handed profession. All of the instruments and equipment we use are for righted-handed surgeons. It is possible to have left-handed instruments, but most leftys find them awkward to use, as they have, for the most part, adapted to the right hand way of life from a very early time.

The main reason for these few words about handedness is to tell those left-handed students in surgery that they should not use this impediment as a crutch. Do not complain about it and do not make excuses for it. It is probably not a good idea to teach yourself to be ambidextrous, as your brain is already too well adjusted to left handedness. Just do the best that you can do, and realize that you are in good company with the likes of Leonardo DaVinci, Beethoven, Michelangelo, Ben Franklin, Isaac Newton, Albert Einstein, Charlie Chaplin, Picasso, and the infamous Jack the Ripper.

Library and Filing System

It is never too early to start building your own, personal library. You have saved some of the important books from medical school, and that is a good start. Books on anatomy and surgical technique should be kept forever. The standard textbooks in surgery are quite expensive but necessary to keep. If there is a particular book that you must have, and cannot afford, you might ask one of the pharmaceutical representatives to purchase it for you. You should ask the industry representatives, whether there are any particular books which they routinely give to residents. Always be on the lookout for antique books and books of historical interest.

Throughout your residency, you will accumulate papers, brochures, handouts, reprints, etc., which most often, will result in stacks of papers and ultimately will end up in the trash. Much of this "stuff" is good to have for reference when the times arise. Start now by purchasing a box of color file folders. Place these documents in appropriately labeled folders, and save them forever. It will make your life a little more orderly. You can easily refer to them when necessary. Some of them will have a historical value in years to come.

Cameras

A camera is a valuable tool for the resident in surgery:

- To document the extent of injuries
- To document appropriate preoperative and intraoperative pathology
- To document postoperative results
- To copy x-rays for presentations
- To assist in Power Point presentations
- To photograph family and friends

For those residents and fellows in the specialties dealing with the surgery of appearance (oral-maxillofacial surgery, otolaryngology-head and neck surgery, plastic surgery), a camera is indispensable and should be carried at all times.

At this writing, approximately seventy five percent of all cameras sold in the US, are digital. There are many digital cameras to choose from and so many variations in option, it will be impossible to sort them out for you in this book. However, you should be aware of some of the important features to look for and learn about.

Consider when purchasing:

- The number of *pixels* generally refers to the final quality of the picture the camera will produce. The more pixels, the less grainy the picture. It is important to realize that there are other factors that contribute to the final quality, such as monitor quality, photographic paper quality, and projector quality. Pixels are expensive, so there is a limit to the number of pixels you should consider purchasing. Most professional photographers believe that for routine medical photography, 3.5 megapixels is all that you need. You will not see the difference in printed or projected work with more than 3.5 megapixels.
- **Digital Zoom vs. Optical Zoom.**
- **Lenses.**
- **Single Lens Reflex** cameras.
- **Batteries** should be at least lithium, rechargeable, and you should always have an extra in your bag.
- **Storage** devices usually consist of minidisks. Most cameras are sold with only a small-sized disk. It will be necessary to purchase a larger one (1 gigabyte) immediately.
- Some cameras have the ability to record **video**. This feature, although not very useful in medicine, is nice to have. A considerable amount of storage (1 gigabyte) permits several minutes of filming in this mode.
- **Software** comes with each camera. Make sure that it is compatible with your computer, fairly easy to use, and that it has a rather comprehensive filing system so that you can appropriately organize the hundreds of pictures that you will take.

- The **display** is a very important feature that deserves mentioning. Not only should it be clear and bright, but it should also swivel so that you can take bird's eye view pictures in the operating room.

Question your attendings and the more senior residents. Ask them what they like and do not like about their cameras.

You should now be getting the idea that purchasing a camera for medical purposes is a very complicated process. In speaking with sales personnel, you will be able to quickly discern if they know what they are talking about. If they do not, then move on to another store. You might try speaking with the photographer on staff at your hospital or university. They are usually very willing to help.

Computers

This is a huge subject, and in another forum, could occupy the space of an entire book. In today's world you must have a computer. Laptop or desktop is up to you. Realize that either will be more than adequate for the needs of most individuals. You should be very discriminating in purchasing this item, and at the same time understand that this will not be the first, second, or even third computer that you will own.

Some things to keep in mind:

- Get the largest screen that you can afford. Flat screens are nice, but cathode ray tubes (CRT) are less expensive, have better picture quality and faster refresh rates. The liquid crystal display (LCD) takes up much less desk space, has a comparable picture, but are more expensive.
- Get the largest hard drive that you can afford.

- Get the most memory that you can afford. Actually, memory affects your speed more than the central processing unit (CPU).
- Do not spend much money on processor speed.
- Make sure that Microsoft Office with Power Point is installed.
- If you are able, you should negotiate to have photo editing software (Adobe Photoshop, Ulead, etc.) installed at no charge to you.
- Printers come in all sizes, shapes, and qualities. They all will do the job, and usually will have to be replaced in one to three years. A laser printer will be more expensive, but may be worth the extra money in the long term. Aside from the higher quality print, a laser printer will print 1000 copies for about the same price as an ink-jet printer will print 100 copies.
- A CD-RW (read/write) is mandatory. A DVD–RW is nice to have.
- Do not fool around with dial-up internet service. Get a DSL or equivalent line, and subscribe to the largest server.
- It is more practical at this stage of your life to buy a name brand computer with matching accessories. It is not a good idea to put together a hybrid computer from a little known manufacturer.

You can spend a lot of time accessorizing your computer setup, but for now, the above suggestions will give you a good start.

Ethics

It appears that there is a slightly different set of ethics for every job, profession, organization, government, and religion. *Medical Ethics* is described as: "The rules or standards governing the conduct of a person or the conduct of the members of a profession." Truly, the principles of medical ethics were set down by Hippocrates in his "oath," and if we carefully dissect it, we will be able to answer almost every ethical question that we will encounter. The problem is that so many of our contemporary ethical dilemmas now require an interpretation, often by a committee, to the exclusion of the more ancient, simple, practical tenants of the code of ethics.

This subject is huge, often overwhelming, and beyond the scope of this book. For more than 155 years, the American Medical Association's *Code of Medical Ethics* has been the standard and most comprehensive guide to physicians on ethics related issues. It is published on their website, and we recommend it to you.

Charity

Interns and residents are a poor bunch, or so they think. In reality, they are right in the middle of monetary compensation in the entire country. We all give in the form of free care or indigent care; that is your duty and privilege. Charity is another story. It does not always mean giving money. There are many ways you can be charitable; however, money is often the most needed method, and the least time-consuming for your busy schedule.

Consider a couple of dollars a week to a charity of your choice. Work at a soup kitchen once a month. Volunteer to the Red Cross or Salvation Army once in a while. There are so many ways to give that you will have no trouble finding them or them finding you. Involve your spouse and your children.

Missions

During your training, you may have the opportunity to participate in a medical mission to some underserved area on this planet. If at all possible, do not pass up these opportunities. In fact, seek them out. Your chief will, most likely, be proud to permit you to go, and you will benefit not only educationally, but with a real sense of having done something good. The expenses of some missions are paid by various agencies. More often than not, you will have to pay.

Political Action Committees

It seems a little distant to think of politics at a time like this in your training, but, as much as we may not approve, both local and national politics is a part of medicine today, and we just have to get used to it. It seems that physicians and politicians do not speak the same language, do not see the same things in their constituencies, and do not have the same goals for healthcare. Today, there are many physicians who hold prestigious positions in our government and who speak for us. It is up to you to continue this medical education of the politicians and to place them in positions of governmental power. Go to the AMA website and educate yourself about this important subject.

Insurance

Money is better than poverty, if only for financial reasons.
—WOODY ALLEN (1935 –)

No matter how rich you become, how famous or powerful, when you die the size of your funeral will still pretty much depend on the weather.
—MICHAEL PRITCHARD

Medical Malpractice Insurance

This will be purchased for you by the hospital. Two important aspects that you should be concerned with are: Is this a *claims-made* or an *occurrence* policy? "Claims made" means that in order to be covered, the claim against you must be filed while you are insured with that company. In other words, when you leave your residency, you are no longer insured for a claim that was made against you during your residency. One remedy for this is to insist that your next insurer provides (usually at no cost) *"tail coverage"*. This will cover you for acts committed during your residency. The other option is for your hospital to buy you an "occurrence" policy. This will cover you by the hospital's insurance company no matter where you are, or when the suit is filed against you.

Another factor in malpractice insurance is the *limits of coverage*. What is the total amount the insurance company will cover? If your net worth is in the millions, this might be a very important number to know. Recent jury awards have been in the tens of millions of dollars.

Unfortunately, all of this is rather moot, as you have little or no say in the type of policy or coverage amount you are given. Nevertheless, you should attempt to educate yourself on these issues, as malpractice insurance will be required for the rest of your career, and you must eventually become an expert on the subject.

Life Insurance

If you are given life insurance as part of your resident's employment package, you should inquire about the possibility of extending it when you leave the institution. The earlier in life you are insured, the less premium you will pay. Also, consider purchasing the insurance for the longest possible time, with a fixed premium that cannot be increased.

It is a good idea to study the types of life insurance before buying it. Yet, do not wait too long, as your premium will only increase. It is wise to be careful, because a lot of insurance sales people are scouting for young doctors.

In general, there are two kinds of individual policies, *whole life* and *term*. A term policy is less expensive and has a fixed annual premium for a certain number of years. The coverage, however, stops when you stop paying the premium, or the certain number of years has expired. A whole life policy is a good way for a young person to be insured. It is more expensive than a term policy, but part of the premium is invested for you, and you benefit from the interest, which is re-invested for you. This interest amount will eventually pay the premiums, year after year. So, if you have been diligent in paying your premiums in the beginning years, you will be insured at no cost in the later years. You may also borrow against the money in your account.

Purchasing life insurance is very important when needed, but everybody does not need it. The entire subject becomes almost a philosophy of life. Most will agree that it should not be considered a lottery winning for the beneficiaries. If you have children and/or your spouse has a good job, they may not need your insurance money. If you have incurred considerable debt, as a result of home loans, car loans, and school loans, insurance money will come in handy for those you leave behind. Remember, life insurance is rather costly, and if it is not necessary, do not buy it. However, before you take this advice, you should check with knowledgeable people. Everybody's situation is different, and the options are endless.

Remember, with life insurance, it pays to start young.

Disability Insurance

Most residency training programs will purchase a small disability insurance policy for you. If you must pay the premium yourself, you should be aware of the following: Make sure you are covered if you are disabled *in your specialty*. Or, you might find yourself disabled to do surgery, but not psychiatry. You will also want to know the time period from when you are totally disabled, to when the checks start arriving. The shorter this lag period, the more the premium. Also, the period of disability covered should last at least until age 64, and premium payment should be suspended during the time of disability.

Usually, the institution-paid-for disability policy is not adequate for the average young professional. You should be able to increase it significantly for a fairly low premium. It could be very worth your while to do that, especially if you have a young family.

Health Care Insurance

No cutting corners here. Get the best you can afford for you and your family. One bad accident or serious illness could break you financially for many years. Be concerned and ask questions about the co-pay, deductibles, prescription drugs, and excluded benefits (like mental illness). The exclusion of mental illness is not acceptable in today's world, where it seems as though more and more doctors are developing addictions, or committing suicide. There is not much you can do about these items short of paying additional premiums. However, it might make sense to consider the expense. You can often opt to add coverage for dental and vision services. They are most often worth the small added expense.

Read your policy carefully for hidden benefits like discounts on eyeglasses, medical devices, medications, etc.

In the years to come, you will become an expert on health care insurance, so start now to understand this evolving subject.

Long-Term Care Insurance

You may be a bit too young to consider long-term care, but again, the younger you are when you buy, the less the premium. It is a good idea to educate yourself on this subject.

Family and Friends

Happiness is having a large, loving, close-knit family in another city.

—George Burns (1896–1996)

Most nonmedical people have not the vaguest idea exactly what you do at the hospital. You bring home a lot of juicy stories, you are tired and irritable, but family and friends are unaware of the intricacies of your job, and the huge commitment you have undertaken. You are seeing many things that few are privy to. Perhaps you are more peaceful with yourself. Life seems to hold a different meaning. It is impossible to be around sickness and disease all day, and not to be affected in many ways. People notice the change that you are going through, but they do not quite understand it. It certainly would not be a bad idea to permit those closest to you (spouse, significant other, mother, etc.) to read this book as an aid to appreciate what you are going through, to understand your commitment both in time and energy, and to help them comprehend your possible mood swings.

Your immediate family is going to suffer during your training. They probably have already come to understand your time obligation. Even at home, you will have little time for family niceties. So, be very cognizant that you are not the only one in distress. Be very jealous of your time with your family and friends. Build that time into your daily and weekly routine, and make it high quality.

A word about "medical secrets" is in order. It is acceptable to tell family and friends about interesting things that happen in the hospital, but be very careful not to be too specific. Breaches in HIPAA (see Chapter 21: HIPAA) can get you fired. Telling stories about your attendings by name or reference, your colleagues, the institution, or the patients can come back at you in ways that you cannot dream of. Although you may seem to be a more interesting person when you tell these stories, remain professional and generic in recounting them.

Your Health

> *Happiness is nothing more than good health*
> *and a bad memory.*
>
> —ALBERT SCHWEITZER

The residency period places unusual demands on your life, both mentally and physically. It is a burden on your entire system and can be truly overwhelming. Unlike the clinic rotations in medical school, you are thrust into the real world of disease, trauma, life and death, and *you* are making the medical decisions. Having this responsibility can be both exhilarating and depressing. These extremes of feelings will eventually lessen with time and experience, but that is not to say that they will or should become blunted. As you learn to internalize and, at will, externalize these feelings, you will develop a healthier mind and more mature compassion.

In an effort to give your mind every opportunity to function correctly, it is mandatory that your body is healthy. You could consciously strengthen your mind or your psyche. However, your body is always at your beck and call, just waiting to be strengthened. When your body is kept in good condition, your mind has less to contend with.

As difficult as it may seem, you should place yourself on a regular *physical fitness program*. Of course you have time. Right! Make the time for fitness, as it is very important for you, your family, and your patients to have not only an intelligent doctor but also one who exemplifies good health. Here are some ideas to get you started:

- If you are already on a program of exercise, continue it.
- Join a fitness center. The hospital often has special prices at a center, and, if associated with a university, it could be free of charge.
- Use the stairs for one to three flights.
- If practical, walk to and from your home.
- Ride a bike to work, on the weekends, or anytime.
- Take long walks. Gradually lengthen your distance to three to four miles a day, three to four times per week.
- Get up a regular basketball, football, or volleyball game.
- Ask somebody to buy you a treadmill.

The important thing is to be consistent in your effort, even when you do not feel like expending much energy.

Residency brings with it a whole new **eating** agenda, and the associated problems of eating too much, not enough, or not correctly. Here are some suggestions:

- If you are grossly overweight, lose weight. Obesity does not engender patient confidence.
- No donuts in the doctors' lounge.

- Try a bagel (no cream cheese) in the morning.
- No fast food. Not even in a pinch. If you must indulge, most fast food places have some dietetic items on the menu.
- Cut down on fat and calories, but do it consistently.
- No fad diets. You cannot afford to take a chance on the metabolic changes they can induce. Consult the hospital dietician.
- No munching in-between meals.

One more health issue is also important. Much of your mental and physical health is determined by how much **fun** you have. Permit yourself the gift of having fun when it is appropriate. This includes time-outs, when you relinquish the trials and tribulations of being in charge of human life. It is cleansing, purifying, and just plain relaxing to regularly be with family and friends, go to a movie, or just take it easy with a good book. It is likewise important to be able to laugh and enjoy it, be humorous and be enjoyed by others.

Dr. Florman's creed:

- Laugh when it's funny.
- Cry when it's sad.
- Joke when appropriate.
- Be serious when being serious is necessary.
- Be happy all of the time. You should be happy; just look at where you are and what you have accomplished.

Vacations

Your vacation time is precious to you. Do not waste a moment of it. Your body and mind depends on period of rest. It should be mandatory to get out of town and do something mindless for a few days a year. There is no intention in this chapter to tell you where to go or what to do; however, with a little study and forethought, you will be able to schedule a vacation like the expert you will become.

The following suggestions will assure you that the planning essentials of your vacation will be done in a timely and complete fashion.

- Negotiate the schedule and coverage with your colleagues. Remember, they will have to pick up the slack.
- Schedule your vacation in writing with the department at least 6 weeks in advance.
- Make sure there are no scheduling conflicts with other residents.
- For obvious reasons, and whether or not it is a rule, do not schedule vacations for the 6-week period beginning July 1, or for the month of June.
- Several people should know how to contact you in case of an emergency. Leave your travel plans and destination phone number with the department secretary, your chief resident and whomever is staying in your home.
- Before you actually leave, call the switchboard and tell them that you will be away, and whom to call in your absence.
- Just before departing, debrief your colleagues about your patients in the hospital as well as any patients with particular problems.
- Complete all of your dictation and medical records.
- Any patient at home with ongoing problems may be told of your departure, and whom to call if necessary.

18

The Transition

Part 2

If you limit your choices only to what seems possible or reasonable, you disconnect yourself from what you truly want, and all that is left is a compromise.

—ROBERT FRITZ

Introduction

Transitioning out of your training program is a complicated and lengthy procedure. This chapter should be read and digested by not only the resident or fellow who is finishing his training, but also by those just beginning their training, as the preparation for this transition really began when you decided to become a surgeon. This is, or will be, the culmination of everything that you have worked so hard for, and your every action should be directed to that day when you will assume the responsibility for making the medical decisions, for where you and your family will live, and precisely how you will want to practice your new skills. Many of the aspects in this decision-making process will evolve quite naturally and automatically as time goes on. Your goals may go through several changes as your ability and mind develops. This is a very healthy process. However, you must start preparing and positioning yourself very early on for the numerous life-changing events that are in store for you.

This section of the book is meant to be only a primer to facilitating your transition from the rather sheltered life of training to the certainly complex life in the real world of medicine. You will have to digest a plethora of information in a short period of time, becoming an expert on subjects which you have not yet heard of. Throughout this necessary ordeal, you must not lose sight of your primary mission: to practice good medicine, take care of your family and yourself, and be a good citizen.

The Start

The practice of surgery is a passion. For some, general surgery satisfies that passion very well, but for others, for one reason or another, a surgical specialty meets the need for fulfillment. For some, the full training in surgery, or one of the surgical specialties, is not enough, and more specialized training can be had in the form of a fellowship. Your choices following residency are numerous:

- Fellowship training
- Private practice
  - Solo
  - Group
    - ✓ Single specialty
    - ✓ Multispecialty
- Academia
- Another specialty
- Retire

Each possibility has many alternatives, which become a matter of investigation and elimination. It is not unusual for a person to choose one route and following analysis, eliminate it and choose another. In reality, there are no rules for choosing. It just seems to come with experience and a great deal of patience.

It is acceptable not to have chosen your final goal early in the process, but some day you will have to weigh all of the variables and reach a firm decision on what you want to do with the rest of your life. So, many factors will determine your decision that it is impossible to advise you in this book. In the end, it is often a very difficult decision to make, and it is one that should never be made by default. In other words, do not choose a less-than-perfect avenue for the future, just because the other avenues may be worse.

You can be assured that your final decision will most likely be correct if once you have made that decision, you stop debating the issue, and put your entire self into your new choice.

Fellowship Training

Fifteen to twenty percent of those completing a residency in surgery will seek additional training in the form of a fellowship. Choosing a certain fellowship position depends on precisely what you are looking for in postgraduate education, who is in charge of the fellowship program, and in what part of the country you want to spend six months or a year. Fellowship should be considered if:

- There is a particular expertise that you want to acquire.
- Your training was deficient in a particular subject.
- You want to bide time while waiting for a practice opportunity.

Fellowships are offered by institutions and by private individuals. Although there are lists of fellowships available, and many of them advertise positions in the journals, the best way to learn about them is from your attendings and your chief. They are able to make recommendations based on their experience and knowledge of the principal individuals in the fellowship programs.

Acceptance to most fellowship programs is highly competitive, and the ACGME matching program does not apply to many of them. You should start the process of applying at the very earliest time permitted. Remember, only the best letters of introduction and recommendation will help you. Telephone calls or candid comments by your chief or attendings will embellish your application.

An interview will certainly be required and will likely be the most important aspect of your application. Be assured, the interviewer will be very experienced and able to pick up on the nuances of every word that you say. Be yourself. Be relaxed. Do not practice answers. Do not brag. Just permit your education and personality to shine through.

This application process must reflect every aspect of your life and persona to date. If you have been an exemplary student, you should not have much trouble seeking the most appropriate fellowship.

Private Practice

Approximately eighty percent of residents and fellows completing their training will choose private practice. Generally, in making this very important decision, you should consider the following two questions, and strictly adhere to their order of importance:

1. Where do You and Your Spouse Want to Live?

This is the most important question, and many factors enter into this decision (i.e., geographical location, climate, schools, family, leisure opportunities, ease of travel to and from that location, homes, etc.) It is essential that your spouse, fiancé, or significant other is in total agreement.

2. Solo, Group, Multispecialty or Clinic?

This decision will be based on the type of person you are; your ultimate goals in the practice of surgery; the opportunities available to you; and whether you desire to be your own boss, work for others, or a combination of the two.

There are many resources available to help you in this decision, notably, the American Medical Association and your specialty society. We cannot advise you as to the type of practice, because of the complexity of the variables and the continuous changes in each possibility. These many factors will become very apparent to you as you begin to sort out what is available.

Considering practice options can begin as early as your first year, but should not occupy much of your thoughts until well into your last year. By January of your last year, you should know where you are going, be comfortable with the people involved, and be far along in the negotiation phase. Always leave ample time and have stand-by options, should these negotiations break down. Under no circumstances should you force yourself into any kind of practice as a last ditch measure.

Generically speaking, preparation for practice opportunities coincides with the beginning of your residency training. All of the things that we have discussed in this book will now embellish your chances of getting the best fellowship, or attracting the most worthy private practices. Or, these same "things" can come back to haunt you. This would be a good time to again read Chapter 1, "The Transition—Part 1". Now, you will have to demonstrate to others, usually outside of your training program, that you are the appropriate choice. You will also have to depend on those in your institution for kind words and helpful suggestions. If there is someone who you did not get along well with, you can be assured that he will be contacted for a candid discussion of your character. Your entire education, your whole persona, and your fondest dreams, all come to this convergence point in time. Repetition is in order:

- Be **honest** (with yourself and others).
- Be **kind** (with yourself and others) (it costs you nothing).
- Be **humble**.
- Be **prepared**.

Academia?

Academic careers can be very satisfying and must be seriously considered when deciding what to do with your life. The rewards are numerous, however they carry a totally different set of problems than private practice.

Pros:
- Intellectually rewarding
- Relatively stable
- Opportunity to advance in rank
- Established practice
- No initial financial obligation
- Interns and residents to assist you
- Research and writing opportunities
- Camaraderie
- Cutting edge in medicine
- Opportunity for innovation
- Coverage
- Large institution benefits
- A good jump-off point to private practice

Cons:

- You are not your own boss
- May not be as financially rewarding
- You do not choose your partners
- You must perform academically to stay in
- Numerous meetings
- A small voice in a large crowd

The Search

Most practice-offers appear fortuitously, but it is up to you to keep your eyes and ears open and take a proactive role in at least superficially investigating all possible practice opportunities. A good place to begin your search is with your attendings and chief. These discussions should take place "by appointment," not in hallways or over the operating table. Knowing your abilities, capabilities, and temperament, they are in the best position to advise you and attempt to match you with an appropriate opportunity.

Continuously monitor the classified advertisements in the periodic journals of your specialty society the Journal of the American Medical Association, the throw-away journals and magazines, and the internet medical bulletin boards. There are booths at the large national meetings and conferences with representatives of companies who make it their business to find jobs for young surgeons. You should make yourself known at each. It is a very good idea to go to at least one national meeting a year (even if you have to pay). This is where you will network for the future. There are medical head-hunters who will eventually seek you out; it is not a good idea to wait for this to happen, as the timing most certainly will not be appropriate.

The Decision

We hope that this will be the last major career decision that you will have to make. Sometimes the decision of what to do following graduation comes very fortuitously, not infrequently with a casual offer of a practice opportunity. Sometimes the same decision-making process is very painful and disruptive to your life. Regardless, it pays to take your time with the process, be thorough in your investigations, and do not get yourself into any situation, or become associated with any person, until you are completely comfortable. At this point, you have not obligated yourself to any definitive decision; that is a long way off. If you are not comfortable with future negotiations, you must courteously go back to your search options and consider this false start as a lesson in business. Once you have come to a tentative conclusion, and there is an offer on the table, it is time to start the rather lengthy, sometimes expensive, always difficult, process of actually making the deal.

The Investigation

To this point, you have done everything correctly, and now it behooves you to expend a considerable amount of effort into meticulously investigating the opportunities you have chosen. This is the most important exercise in the process. An offer has been made, albeit casual and in general terms. Much discussion has occurred, and you and your future partner (practitioner, group, university, clinic, hospital) have agreed in principal that you are, or could be, compatible, have similar goals, thoughts of practice, ethics, work principles, and that now you should proceed with the details. The verbal agreements that you have both made should now be put into a formal written contract. Read it carefully. It should agree in essence with all that you have discussed. If it does not, you must call your future partner and iron out the problems. This is best done by telephone, not e-mail. If the major points of contention cannot be worked out, then it is time to respectfully and hastily begin looking for another opportunity. If the issues are minor, then work them out. Remember, a good partnership is like a good marriage; give and take.

Once the contract looks good, you must take it to an attorney of your choosing who is very familiar with employment contracts for physicians. He will dissect it, explain to you the possible pitfalls, and probably rewrite parts of it. He may even reinvent it to the point where it becomes untenable to your future partner. Attorneys have a tendency to make contracts so correct that the human and practical elements become secondary. It will be up to you, in consultation with your attorney, to decide what is important to you and worth the fight, and what is not important or not worth making issues which could only antagonize.

A "non-compete" clause will most likely be included in any contract that you receive. It will be better if you can negotiate your way out of it, or at least have it wear off after a reasonable period of time, such as one year. Non-competes (sometimes called "covenant not to compete") protects the principle entity from you gathering his or her practice and going into competition across the street. Once signed, they are very difficult and usually impossible to revoke. Most states will uphold a non-compete clause under any circumstance, and most contracts will contain one. For this reason, it is good to take your time, and be as sure as you are able that this proposed partnership is right for you.

Additional items that must be addressed and carefully evaluated in a contract will be:

- Remuneration
- Term of the contract
- Buy-ins, buy-outs
- Partnership tract
- Malpractice insurance (do not forget tail coverage)
- Disability insurance
- Life insurance
- Expense apportioning
- Work apportioning
- Vacations
- Exit from practice strategies for you and for your partner

Some items that may not be part of the contract but are important to know:

- Staff support and who pays for it
- Auto lease or expense
- Signage
- Marketing expenses
- Routine inspection of the accounting books

In the short space of this book, it is difficult to identify all of the idiosyncrasies of a contract between doctors, or between doctors and entities. We can only say that there are many, and that professional, unemotional, detached help is required.

Due Diligence

Before signing on the dotted line, it is a good idea to take a time-out for a few days to three or four weeks and to just:

- Reflect on what you have accomplished.
- Compare your dreams to the realities that are about to take place.
- Assure yourself that you are not just settling for second best.

- Make sure that the lofty goals that you have set for yourself will be satisfied.
- Be peaceful that you are making the correct decisions for your present and future families.

Obligations

This chapter on transitions would not be complete without reminding you of your departing obligations to your present training program. Here is a quick checklist:

- Work until the last day.
- Do not save your vacations until June.
- Make sure your dictations are up to date.
- Visit the medical records department just prior to the end.
- Leave your forwarding home phone number, business phone number, fax number, cellular number, home address, and business address with the department secretary.
- Clean out your locker, and return the key to the proper person.
- Make a special point of going around the hospital and thanking people who have been a part of your life on your way up.
- Say a special farewell and thank you to your chief and your attendings. Ask them if you may communicate with them in the future.

The Beginning

Your mentors have finished instructing you in the fine art of surgery, and how to behave as a surgeon. The rest is up to you. There are no books to show you how to comport yourself in practice. On June 30, you were a resident or fellow. On July 1, all of a sudden you are a surgeon. Very simply, you only need to practice the principles of surgery that you have learned, and strictly adhere to the basic rules: be honest, be humble, be kind, and be prepared. Oh yes, there are now two more rules: be proud and be happy.

19

The Mentor's Wrap-Up

I imagine the life of a surgeon can be very rewarding...
Obviously you have saved the lives of many people...
Is that what led you to become a surgeon?
No, I just liked the little green booties!

—PEANUTS

Mentoring students, interns, and residents in surgery is an enriching, enlightening, and satisfying avocation, made possible to only a few of us fortunate enough to be permitted to work with today's bright and dedicated surgeons of the future. I am certain that I may take the liberty of speaking for all of us mentors, and for you as well, the mentors of tomorrow, who will be the standard torchbearers of learning, teaching, research, and practicing the flower of medicine—surgery.

What follows is the essence of this book. Live by these doctrines, and you will certainly be the pride of our profession:

- You owe a debt of gratitude to each of your patients; good, bad, kind, evil, young, old, clean, dirty, friendly, mean, happy, angry, calm, violent. If it was not for them, you would have nobody to learn from. Somehow, in some way, you must show your gratitude.

- Have great respect for your teachers; all of them, even the ones you do not like or trust. You learn something from every one of them.
- Never fail to pay attention to your parents, siblings, spouse, children, and friends. It makes you a better person.
- Make every effort to stay healthy in your body and mind.
- Keep humor in every aspect of your life. *On the subject of "joking around" about patients, a famous neurosurgeon lamented to me one day that his specialty exposed him to unimaginable and incomparable human tragedies and experiences. When he would find himself laughing or joking at something that was really not funny, he would tell those around him that it was not out of disrespect, ignorance, or malice, but that the only other option was to internalize it and then go home and spend the rest of the day and night in his closet.*
- Be compassionate to your patients, to your very soul.

The following aphorisms were compiled by the late Dr. Eugene Kilgore, a hand surgeon, and are known as Kilgoreisms. They are very salient today:

- You can take a lifetime to establish a reputation, and lose it in a day.
- Think, "us," "our," not "me," "I."
- Think, "What can I do to help," not, "That is not my job."
- You have to give to get.
- Do not be reluctant to say, "I do not know."
- Be willing to learn from everyone, especially your patients.

- Run it by one who has been there before, especially if he/she has gray hairs.
- Technique comes naturally, or is rapidly learned by most, but judgment takes time and experience.
- Seasoned judgment is the cumulative product of episodes of bad judgment.
- Do not hesitate to delegate to a subordinate colleague, and in them never be intolerant of honest mistakes.
- Responsibility brings out the best in anyone, and breeds early maturity.
- Only do for your patients, what you would be willing to have done for yourself.
- Beware of advising "Nothing else has worked, so we had better operate."
- Surgery is *injury*.
- Do not practice by intimidation.
- You do not own your patient.
- Encourage a second opinion.
- If a patient would rather go to someone else, encourage it.
- Do not belittle the previous practitioner. Remember that you, too, are not perfect.
- Simplicity is predictable, complexity is not.
- If you let patients have sufficient time to tell you in detail what is wrong and how it came about, you will find out what ails them and determine what to do for them.
- Do not be a cookbook physician and surgeon. Improvise and adapt.
- Practice good medicine, not defensive medicine.
- Keep detailed records.
- All patients are not created equally, but all count equally.
- Do not be complacent. Your reputation rests on the success of your treatment of your last patient.

- The greatest sin is rationalization of avoidable errors and crimes of omission and commission.
- Practice medicine as an art, not a science.
- Keep skid chains on your tongue; always say less than you think. How you say it often counts more than what you say.
- Never let an opportunity pass to say a kind and encouraging thing to or about somebody. Praise good work done, regardless of who did it. If criticism is needed, criticize helpfully, never spitefully.
- Be interested in others, in their pursuits, their welfare, their homes and families. Let everyone you meet know that you regard him/her as one of importance.
- Be cheerful. Keep the corners of your mouth turned up. Hide your pains, worries and disappointments under a smile. Laugh at good stories and learn to tell them.
- Preserve an open mind on all debatable questions. Discuss, but not argue. It is a mark of superior minds to disagree and yet be friendly.
- Let your virtues speak for themselves and refuse to talk of another's vices. Make it a rule to say nothing of another unless it is something good.
- Be careful of another's feelings. Wit and humor at the other fellow's expense are rarely worth the effort.
- Pay no attention to ill-natured remarks about you. Be assured that nobody will believe them. Disordered nerves and a bad digestion are common causes of backbiting.
- Do not be too anxious about your dues. Do your work, be patient, and keep your disposition sweet. Forget self and you will be rewarded.

Being a mentor is not difficult, and in fact takes no effort at all. One only needs to selflessly impart Dr. Kilgore's knowledge in a gracious way to an eager student. So, who gets more out of it, the mentor or the mentoree? The answer lies with Dr. Kilgore's final piece of advice:

The road to success lies in meeting responsibility with an open inquisitive mind, imagination, and hard work, tempered with humility, kindness, fidelity, time for play, the arts, family, as well as a good laugh. The lasting measure of success is how much remains after you have gone, that continues to be of value to others.

Commonly Used Web Sites

Medicine In General

World Health Organization	www.who.org
Center for Disease Control	www.cdc.gov
National Library of Medicine (Medline)	www.nlm.nih.gov
WebMD	www.webmd.com
Mdlinx	www.mdlinx.com
Ovid (Journals on line, through library)	www.ovid.com
HIPAA information	http://www.hhs.gov/ocr/hipaa/
Joint Commission on Accreditation Of Hospitals	www.JCAHO.org

Surgery

Accreditation Council for Graduate Medical Education	www.acgme.org
American College of Surgeons	www.facs.org
Association of Academic Surgery	www.aasurg.org
The Association for Surgical Education	www.surgicaleducation.com
The American Board of Surgery	www.absurgery.org
Association of Women Surgeons	www.womensurgeons.org
Am. Soc. of Colon and Rectal Surgeons	www.facrs.org
Am. Soc. of Breast Surgeons	www.breastsurgeons.org
Am. Soc. of Plastic Surgery	www.plasticsurgery.org
Am. Soc. of Surgical Oncology	www.surgonc.org

Society of Thoracic Surgeons	www.sts.org
Am. Soc. of Transplant Surgeons	www.asts.org
Am. College of Obstetrics and Gynecology	www.acog.org
Am. Academy of Orthopedic Surgeons	www.aaos.org
Am. Assoc. of Neurological Surgeons	www.neurosurgery.org

PDA

Free Palm programs	www.Freewarepalm.com
Downloadable medical	www.PDAmd.com
Downloadable medical	www.epocrates.com
Free news	www.avantgo.com

Finance

Motley Fool	www.fool.com
Charles Schwab	www.schwab.com
Silicon Investor	wwww.siliconinvestor.com
Yahoo Financial	www. Yahoo.com

Appendix B

Books of Interest

Surgery

Principles of Surgery, 8th Edition, Seymour I. Schwartz, et al., 2004, McGraw Hill Text.
>   *Principles of Surgery: Companion Handbook*
>   *Principles of Surgery: Pretest and Self-Assessment*
>   *Principles of Surgery: Pretest and Self-Assessment CD ROM*

Basic Surgery, 5th Edition, Hiram C. Polk, Jr., Bernard Gardner, H. Harlan Stone, 1995, Quality Medical Publishing, Inc.

Textbook of Surgery: The Biological Basis of Modern Surgical Practice, 16th Edition, David Sabiston and H.Kym Lyerly, 2000, W.B. Saunders.

Textbook of Surgery: Pocket Companion.

Textbook of Surgery: The Biological Basis of Modern Surgical Practice CD Rom.

Surgery: Scientific Principles & Practice, 3rd Edition, Lazar J. Greenfield, 2001, Lippincott, Williams & Wilkins Publishers.

Current Surgical Therapy, 6th Edition, John Cameron, 1998, BC Decker.

Current Surgical Diagnosis and Treatment, 10th Edition, Lawrence Way, 2001, Appleton & Lange.

Trauma: Clinical Care & Pathophysiology, Hiram C. Polk, Jr., J. David Richardson, Louis M. Flint, 1987, Year Book Medical Publishers, Inc.

Atlases

Atlas of Surgical Operations, 8th Edition, Robert Zollinger, 2003, McGraw-Hill.

Atlas of General Surgery, David Sabiston Jr., 1993, WB Saunders, Inc.

Mastery of Surgery, 3rd Edition, Nyhus & Baker, 1996, Little, Brown & Co.

Maingot's Abdominal Operations Volumes I & II, 10th Edition, Michael Zinner, 1997, Appleton & Lange.

Operative Strategy in General Surgery: An Explosive Atlas, 2nd Edition, Jameson L. Chassin, 1994, Springer-Verlag.

Atlas of Laparoscopic Surgery, Garth Ballantyne, 2000, W.B. Saunders, Inc.

Surgical Anatomy and Technique: A Pocket Manual, 2nd Edition, John Skandalakis et al., 2000, Springer-Verlag, Inc.

Handbooks

The Mont Reid Surgical Handbook, 4th Edition, Scott Berry et al., 1997, Mosby Yearbook, Inc.

Handbook of Surgical Intensive Care: Practices of the Surgery Residents at the Duke University Medical Center, 5th Edition, Bryan M. Clary et al., 2000, Mosby Yearbook, Inc.

Abernathy's Surgical Secrets, 4th Edition, Alden H. Harken, 2000, Mosby Yearbook, Inc.

Surgical Recall and Advanced Surgical Recall, Lorne H. Blackbourne, 1997, Williams & Wilkins.

When to Refer to a Surgeon, Susan Galandiuk, 2001, Quality Medical Publishing, Inc.

The Internet for Surgeons, Jeff W. Allen, 2002, Springer-Verlag

Resources

Selected Readings in Surgery, University of Texas Southwestern Medical Center, Monthly subscription.

The Art of Surgical Technique, Milton T. Edgerton, 1988, Williams & Wilkins.

The Physiologic Basis of Surgery, 3rd Edition, J. Patrick O'Leary, editor, 1996, Williams & Wilkins.

Surgical Decision Making, 4th Edition, Lawrence Norton et al., 2000, W.B. Saunders, Inc.